Leadership and Management in Nursing Practice and Education

Leadership and Management in
Nursing Practice and Education

Leadership and Management in Nursing Practice and Education

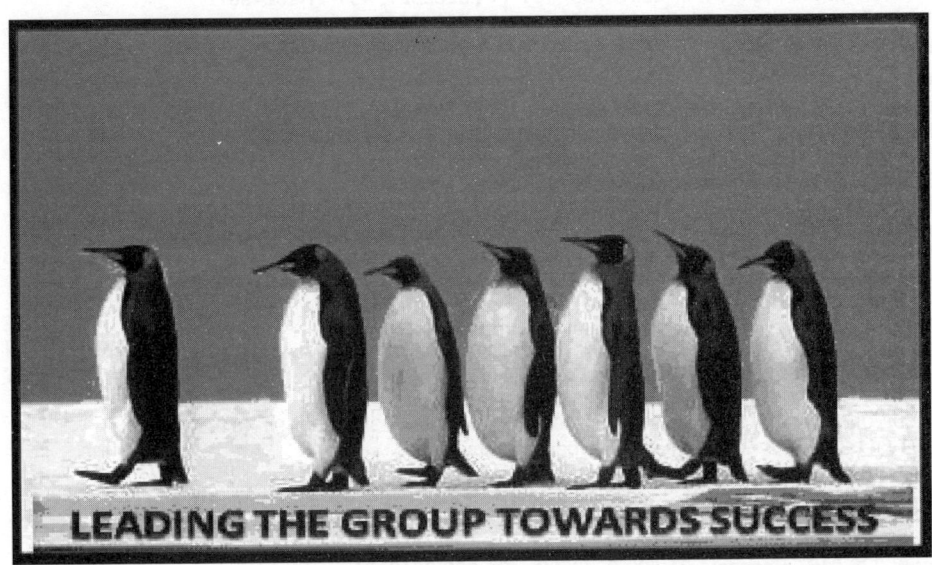

Rebecca Samson
MSc (N) PhD (N)
Professor and HOD of Community Health Nursing
Principal, Padmashree College of Nursing
Bengaluru, India

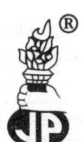

JAYPEE BROTHERS MEDICAL PUBLISHERS (P) LTD

New Delhi • Ahmedabad • Bengaluru • Chennai • Hyderabad • Kochi
Kolkata • Lucknow • Mumbai • Nagpur
St Louis (USA)

Published by
Jitendar P Vij
Jaypee Brothers Medical Publishers (P) Ltd

Corporate Office
4838/24, Ansari Road, Daryaganj, **New Delhi** 110 002, India
Phone: +91-11-43574357

Registered Office
B-3, EMCA House, 23/23B Ansari Road, Daryaganj, **New Delhi** 110 002, India
Phones: +91-11-23272143, +91-11-23272703, +91-11-23282021, +91-11-23245672
Rel: +91-11-32558559   Fax: +91-11-23276490, +91-11-23245683
e-mail: jaypee@jaypeebrothers.com   Visit our website: www.jaypeebrothers.com

Branches

- 2/B, Akruti Society, Jodhpur Gam Road Satellite
  Ahmedabad 380 015   Phones: +91-79-26926233, Rel: +91-79-32988717
  Fax: +91-79-26927094, e-mail: ahmedabad@jaypeebrothers.com
- 202 Batavia Chambers, 8 Kumara Krupa Road, Kumara Park East
  Bengaluru 560 001   Phones: +91-80-22285971, +91-80-22382956, +91-80-22372664
  Rel: +91-80-32714073 Fax: +91-80-22281761   e-mail: bangalore@jaypeebrothers.com
- 282 IIIrd Floor, Khaleel Shirazi Estate, Fountain Plaza, Pantheon Road
  Chennai 600 008   Phones: +91-44-28193265, +91-44-28194897, Rel: +91-44-32972089
  Fax: +91-44-28193231,   e-mail: chennai@jaypeebrothers.com
- 4-2-1067/1-3, 1st Floor, Balaji Building, Ramkote Cross Road
  Hyderabad 500 095   Phones: +91-40-66610020, +91-40-24758498   Rel:+91-40-32940929
  Fax:+91-40-24758499,   e-mail: hyderabad@jaypeebrothers.com
- No. 41/3098, B & B1, Kuruvi Building, St. Vincent Road
  Kochi 682 018, Kerala   Phones: +91-484-4036109, +91-484-2395739, +91-484-2395740
  Fax: +91-844-2395740, e-mail: kochi@jaypeebrothers.com
- 1-A Indian Mirror Street, Wellington Square
  Kolkata 700 013   Phones: +91-33-22651926, +91-33-22276404, +91-33-22276415
  Rel: +91-33-32901926 Fax: +91-33-22656075,   e-mail: kolkata@jaypeebrothers.com
- Lekhraj Market III, B-2, Sector-4, Faizabad Road, Indira Nagar
  Lucknow 226 016   Phones: +91-522-3040553, +91-522-3040554
  Fax: +91-522-3040553, e-mail: lucknow@jaypeebrothers.com
- 106 Amit Industrial Estate, 61 Dr SS Rao Road, Near MGM Hospital, Parel
  Mumbai 400012   Phones: +91-22-24124863, +91-22-24104532, Rel: +91-22-32926896
  Fax: +91-22-24160828, e-mail: mumbai@jaypeebrothers.com
- "KAMALPUSHPA" 38, Reshimbag, Opp. Mohota Science College, Umred Road
  Nagpur 440 009 (MS) Phone: Rel: +91-712-3245220, Fax: +91-712-2704275
  e-mail: nagpur@jaypeebrothers.com

USA Office
1745, Pheasant Run Drive, Maryland Heights (Missouri), MO 63043, USA
Ph: 001-636-6279734   e-mail: jaypee@jaypeebrothers.com, anjulav@jaypeebrothers.com

Leadership and Management in Nursing Practice and Education

© 2009, Rebecca Samson

All rights reserved. No part of this publication should be reproduced, stored in a retrieval system, or transmitted in any form or by any means: electronic, mechanical, photocopying, recording, or otherwise, without the prior written permission of the author and the publisher.

> This book has been published in good faith that the material provided by author is original. Every effort is made to ensure accuracy of material, but the publisher, printer and author will not be held responsible for any inadvertent error(s). In case of any dispute, all legal matters are to be settled under Delhi jurisdiction only.

First Edition: **2009**

ISBN 978-81-8448-462-5

Typeset at   JPBMP typesetting unit
Printed at   Rajkamal Electric Press, B-35/9, G.T.Karnal Road, Delhi-33

Dedicated to
my beloved parents who are my inspiration

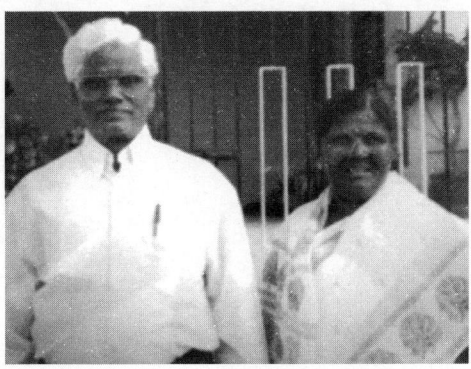

Sri Guduri Joseph and Smt Guduri Vijayamma

Preface

This textbook is designed to highlight the concepts, theories and principles of leadership and management in nursing practice and education.

It introduces the steps of management process and leadership styles which would enable the nursing students/personnel to develop an insight to provide quality care and education in any health care and medical centres in the country to suit the societal needs. It also provides comprehensiveness in understanding the role of a nurse as a Manager.

This book also helps the undergraduate and postgraduate students as well as novice teachers to acquire skills in planning and implementing the curriculum. The guidelines given will serve in the preparation of course materials to teach and evaluate the students in classrooms and also the clinical settings in an effective manner. It helps the teacher to set high level of standards in integrating quality in education and practice.

On the whole, the book provides an access to understand the process of management in nursing practice, health care agencies and nursing education in a comprehensive manner.

Rebecca Samson

Contents

PART A: GENERAL PRINCIPLES OF MANAGEMENT

Unit I: Introduction of Concepts and Principles

01. Definitions and Concepts of Leadership and Management 3
02. Steps in Management Process 7

Unit II: Theories

03. Management Theories 11
04. Leadership Theories 21

Unit III: Leadership Styles

05. Types of Leaders and Leadership Styles 29
06. Time Management 37
07. Communication and Critical Thinking in Management 43
08. Group Dynamics 50

PART B: MANAGEMENT OF NURSING PRACTICE IN HEALTH CARE AGENCIES

Unit IV: Planning

09. Planning Process 55
10. Decision Making and Problem Solving 59
11. Budgeting 62

Unit V: Organizing

12. Systems Theory and Systems Analysis 65
13. Organizational Structure 70

Unit VI: Patient Care Management

14. Management of Hospital Departments 74
15. Management of Nursing Services 83

Unit VII: Personnel Management—Directing

16. Staffing 98
17. Scheduling/Duty Roster 102
18. Job Description 106

19. Performance Appraisal 108
20. Staff Motivation 113
21. Staff Development 118

Unit VIII: Controlling

22. Quality Assurance (QA) 124
23. Ethics in Managing Health Care 131
24. Documentation—Records and Reports 133
25. Change Process—Planned Change 142

PART C : MANAGEMENT OF NURSING EDUCATIONAL INSTITUTIONS

Unit IX: Program Planning

26. Development of Program Objective 149
27. Trends and Issues in Nursing Curriculum Development 154

Unit X: Planning and Organization of Curriculum

28. Curriculum Planning 160
29. Planning and Organization of Clinical Learning Experiences 169

Unit XI: Evaluation System

30. Evaluation in Education—Qualities of Measuring Instruments 178
31. Test Construction and Item Analysis 182
    Appendices *191*
    Glossary *203*
    Index *207*

Part A: General Principles of Management

Unit I: Introduction of concepts and principles

01 Definitions and Concepts of Leadership and Management

OBJECTIVES

1. Describe the terms of leadership and management.
2. Differentiate the concepts of leadership and management.
3. Discuss the characteristics of a leader and manager.
4. Identify the types of power and its influence on a leader/manager.
5. Analyze the relationship between authority and power and relate it to leadership and management.

INTRODUCTION

Nursing is a dynamic and multidisciplinary profession developed through,
- Competencies in nursing skills.
- Interpersonal relations.
- Problem solving and critical thinking.
- The understanding of leadership and management process.

THE PRIMARY PURPOSE OF LEADERSHIP AND MANAGEMENT IS TO WORK TOGETHER WITH OTHER HEALTH TEAM MEMBERS

Definitions

Leadership

Leadership is defined as the **process of influencing others toward a goal** (Bennie and Nanas, 1985).

Effective leaders are those who are capable of obtaining the cooperation and resources needed to achieve their goals.

Management

Leadership and Management are closely related.

Like leadership, **Management** also is a process of influencing others with specific intention of getting them to perform effectively and contributing to meet the organizational goals (Dmker, 1967).

So, management is a process of getting work done through other people.

Who is a leader?

A leader is an influential person have the ability to lead a group or department without having a formal appointment.

Who is a manager?

A manager is formally and officially responsible for the work of a given group.

For example, nurse manager of an unit, or Nursing officer/Director or Dean/ Principal of a college and Medical Superintendent of a hospital, etc.

They are officially responsible to ensure that the unit accomplishes its tasks well.

What a manager must possess in order to fulfill his role?

To fulfill this role.... Managers must possess.
Broader knowledge and skills in the following areas.

- Budgeting
- Planning
- Management theories
- Organizational structure
- Communication skills
- Rules and regulations of agencies
  For example, Health care system/ Educational institutions
- Staff development
- Staff appraisal

Similarities and differences between the leader and the manager

Leader	Manager
• May or may not have an official appointment	• Appointed officially to the position
• Have the power and authority to enforce decisions as long as followers are willing to be lead	• Have power and authority to enforce decisions
• Influence others either formally or informally	• Carry out predetermined policies, rules and regulations
• Interested in risk-taking and exploring new ideas	• Maintain an orderly, controlled, rational and equitable structure
• Relate to people personally in an empathetic manner	• Relate to people according to their roles
• Feel rewarded from personal achievements	• Feel rewarded when fulfilling organizational goals or mission
• May or may not be successful as manager	• They are managers as long as they hold the appointment

Concepts Related to Leadership and Management

A. General Concepts

- Management is a formal, specifically designated position within the organization.
- To be a good manager ....It is absolutely necessary to be an effective leader.

- In fact all nurses should at times assume some leadership roles, but not every one needs to be a manager.
- The difference between leadership and management is equated to effectiveness and efficiency.

B. Specific Concepts

1. Authority and Power
2. Effectiveness and Efficiency

Specific concepts	Emphasis
Authority	It is the legitimate right given to a manager or a leader by an organization in order to command subordinates and to act in the interest of an organization to achieve its goals.
Power	Power is to influence others to act, and it is the most important ingredient of a leader or manager in an organization. It is the ability to impose the will on others to bring about certain behaviors.
Effectiveness	It is related to leadership, vision, and judgment.
Efficiency	It is related to management and mastering routines.

So in any organization authority and power must be given proportionately to carry out the responsibilities. It is the legitimate right to give commands to act in the interest of an organization.

Power is the ability to impose the will on others to bring about certain behaviors in others. There are different types of power which need to be exercised by a leader or manager (Fig. 1.1).

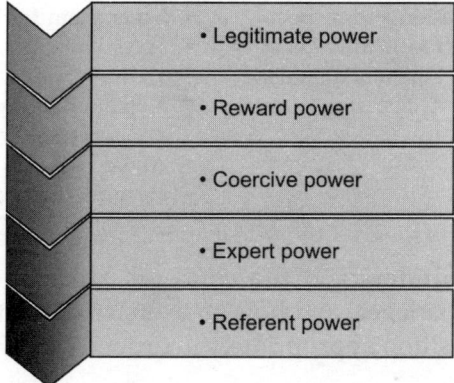

Fig. 1.1: Types of power

Power and Influence in a Leader/Manager

The leader/manager need to use the power given to him by an organization in an appropriate manner depending on the situation.

Types of power	Basis	How to use the power
a. Legitimate power	Given by an organization according to the position. E.g.: Principal/Nursing Directer	• Make polite requests • Use clear and simple language • Explain the reason • Follow-up to check compliance.
b. Reward power	Incentives the leader can provide for the subordinates and value by the group	• Do not over emphasis incentives • Rein force good behavior, don't bribe • Size of the reward should reflect total performance • Money is not only the reward, other means of appreciations may be used. E.g.: Awards, certificates, etc.
c. Coercive power	Found in fear. E.g.: Oral or written warnings; suspension and termination	• Avoid it except when absolutely needed • Determine genuine fault • Discipline promptly without favoritism • State warnings without hostility • Fit the punishment to the seriousness of the fault • Warn before punishing.
d. Expert power	Special ability, skills and knowledge by virtue of education and experience. E.g.: Mastery over the subject and emotional stability	• Avoid careless decisions, rash statements • Keep abreast with current developments • Remain calm in crisis and act confidently • Respect staff ideas and include them • Do not threaten staff self esteem, respect staff concern and explain why the change is needed
e. Referent power	Admiration and respect the staff feels towards a leader. Personal qualities influence charisma.	• Treat them fairly • Avoid hostility, rejection distrust, and indifference • Explain reliance on staff support and cooperation. • Make requests reasonable • Be a good role model.

So, it is essential to understand the concepts, differences and the similarities between a leader and a manager, and how to exercise the authority given to a person according to his or her position appropriately in order to analyze the kind of leadership and be successful.

02 Steps in Management Process

OBJECTIVES

1. List the steps in management process.
2. Describe the process of management.
3. Identify and differentiate various theories in the management.
4. Apply the principles of management theories by the potential young leaders of nursing.

INTRODUCTION

A process is a series of steps or actions which lead to achieve a goal, and it is dynamic. Nurses are familiar with the application of nursing process such as assessing, diagnosing, planning, implementing and evaluating the patient care in the health care management of their patients/clients in any setting. Similarly, nurse leaders must also be aware of various steps involved in the management process.

Generally, the students are aware of managing their learning activities during their professional carrier, and in their work in professional practice. Some of the individuals basically organized but some will learn through exposure to certain situations during their practice. The effective nurses are those who really understand and consciously apply the principles of management to practice.

What is management process?

The management process is like nursing process which include:
- Gathering data from different sources.
- Diagnosing the problems by analyzing the data carefully.
- Plan appropriate actions according to priorities.
- Carry out the interventions suitable.
- Evaluate the out comes of interventions.
- Replan until the identified problems are resolved.

As said in the previous chapter the management is the process of getting work done through others.

Nursing Management

It is the process of working through nursing personnel to promote and maintain health, prevent illness and suffering. The role of nurse manager is to plan, organize, direct, and control available resources in order to provide effective economic care to groups of clients efficiently.

In reality the management process is more complex than nursing process as it directly deals with the management of working with human beings, physical resources, organizational and psychological process within a creative and innovative climate for the realization of organizational goals.

So management is a dynamic process which is universal and can be used in variety of settings and situations.

Henry Fayol (1925) first identified the functions of management as.
- Planning
- Organization
- Command
- Coordination
- Control

Later Luther Gullick (1937) expanded these activities by introducing two more activities in addition. **Planning, Organizing, Staffing, Directing, Co-coordinating, Reporting and Budgeting (POSDECORB).**

All these are again reorganized by clubbing reporting and coordinating under the component of control and classified as five major elements or steps in the management process.

The major five elements of management process as shown in Fig. 2.1.

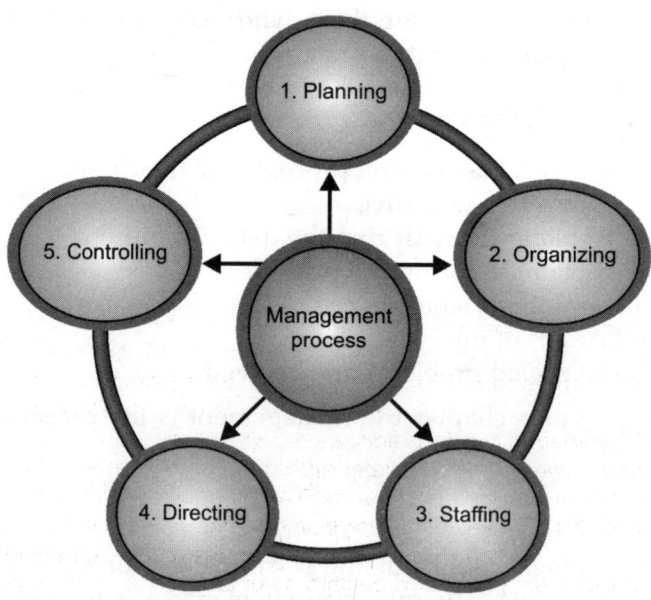

Fig. 2.1: Management process

Planning

"Planning is preparing a blue print"

Planning refers to thinking a head of time and formulation of preliminary thoughts. In other words :

It is a continuous, intellectual process of determining philosophy, objectives, policies, procedures and rules and standards, long- and short-term projected out comes and fiscal course of actions and managing planned change. This is the preliminary and most important step of management process.

Organizing

It is establishing the structure to carry out the plans. Determining the most appropriate type of patient care delivery in a health agency. Or educational programs in an institution. In simple it is **Grouping** the activities to meet its goals.

Other functions involve:

- Working within the structure of an organization,
- Understanding, and
- Using power and authority appropriately.

Staffing

It is a process of assigning competent people to fill the appropriate nursing roles in an institution, designated for the organizational structure through:

- Recruitment and selection of staff,
- Hiring and orienting staff,
- Staff scheduling, and
- Staff development activities.
  Staffing often becomes part of organizing.

Example

Appointment of a Dean for the college of nursing, nursing superintendent for a hospital or a head nurse for a hospital unit, etc.

Directing

Is a process of involving many human resource management responsibilities such as:

- Motivating,
- Managing a conflict,
- Communicating,
- Facilitating, collaborating and coordinating the team.

Controlling

It is an ongoing process to ensure that the activities of an institution or organization adhere to the plan. It includes:
- Quality assurance,
- Performance appraisal,
- Fiscal accountability,
- Legal, ethical and professional control.

An effective manager uses the management process to achieve agency goals through group efforts and follows a predetermined plan in directing employees.

The overall plan for the nursing department is developed jointly by nurses from all hierarchial levels. They specify what needs to be done, how and by whom the responsibilities to be carried out considering the available resources like material, money and man power resources.

Unit II: Theories

03 Management Theories

OBJECTIVES

1. Identify and differentiate various theories in the management.
2. Differentiate various theories and the emphasis made in each theory.
3. Discuss the implications to nursing management.
4. Apply the principles of management theories by the potential young leaders of nursing.

INTRODUCTION

The knowledge on theories of management for nurse leaders can be useful in creating and developing their own management styles. One needs to understand that no single theory can be well fit and guide nursing leaders in every situation. In this chapter some of the important theories developed at different periods of time are discussed in order to help nurse managers to adapt and function effectively.

The four important theories focused for nurse managers are shown in Fig. 3.1.

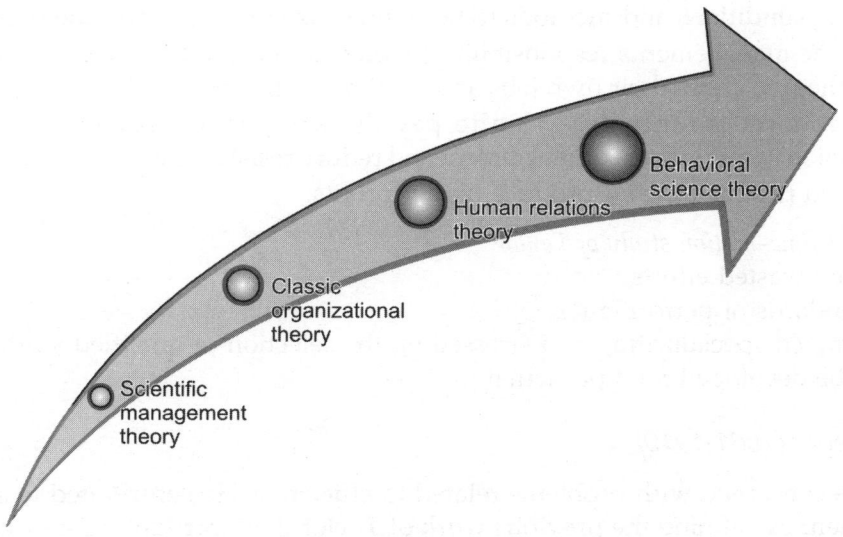

Fig. 3.1: Important theories for nurse managers

SCIENTIFIC MANAGEMENT

Principles

The scientific management focuses on:
- Observation and
- The measurement of outcome

The pioneers of scientific management are:
1. Frederick W. Taylor (1856-1915)
2. Gantt Henry l. Gantt (1861-1919)
3. Emerson (1853-1936)

Taylor's Theory (1856-1915)

Taylor is recognized as father of scientific management. He conducted Time – and – Motion studies to time the workers, analyze their movements and set their standards. He used stop watches. He applied the principles of observation, measurement and scientific comparison to determine the **most efficient** way to accomplish a task.

Achievements of Taylor:
1. He trained his workers to follow the time to complete the task given. The most productive workers were hired even when they were paid an incentive or wage.
2. Labor costs per unit were reduced as a result.
3. Responsibilities of management were separated from the functions of the workers.
4. Developed a systematic approach to determine the most efficient means of production.
5. He considered management function is to plan.
6. Working conditions and methods to be standardized to maximize the production.
7. It was the managements responsibility to select and train the workers rather than allow them to chose their own jobs and train by themselves.
8. He introduced an incentive plan to pay the workers according to the rate of production to minimize workers dissent and reduce resistance to improved methods.
9. Increased production and produce higher profits.

The effect of time–motion study of Taylor
- Reduced wasted efforts
- Set standards of performance
- Encouraged specialization and stressed on the selection of qualified workers who could be developed for a particular job.

Gantt Theory (1861-1919)

Gantt was concerned with problems related to efficiency. He contributed to scientific management by refining the previous work of Taylor than introducing new concepts.

1. He studied the amount of work planned or completed on one axis to the time needed or taken to complete a task on the other axis.
2. Gantt also developed a task and bonus remuneration plan where by workers received a guaranteed day's wages plus a bonus for production above the standard to stimulate higher performance.
3. Gantt recommended to select workers scientifically and provided with detailed instructions for their tasks.
4. He argued for a more Humanitarian approach by management, placing emphasis on service rather than profit objectives.
5. He recognized useful non-monetary incentives such as job security and encouraging staff development.

Emerson's Theory (1853-1936)

His Emphasis was on conservation and organizational goals and objectives.
He defined principles of efficiency related to:

1. Interpersonal relations and to system in management.
2. Goals and ideas should be clear and well-defined as the primary objective is to produce the best product as quickly as possible at minimal expense.
3. Changes should be evaluated-management should not ignore "commonsense" by assuming that big is necessarily better.
4. "Competent counsel" is essential.

His theory explains about

- Management can strengthen discipline or adherence to the rules by justice, or equal enforcement on all records, including adequate, reliable and immediate information about the expenses of equipment and personnel should be available as a basis for decisions.
- Dispatching or production scheduling is recommended.
- Standardized schedules, conditions and written instructions should be there to facilitate performance.
- "Efficiency rewards" should be given for successful completion of tasks.
- Emerson moved further beyond scientific management to classic organizational theory.

CLASSIC ORGANIZATION THEORY

Importance of classic organization theory:

- The classic administration – organization thinking began to receive attention in 1930.
- Organization is viewed as whole rather than focusing solely in production.
- The concepts of scalar levels, span of control, authority, responsibility, accountability, line staff relationships, decentralization, and departmentalization became prevalent.

There are three pioneers who concentrated on classic organization theory.
1. Henry Fayol (1841-1925)
2. Max Webber (1864-1920)
3. James Mooney (1884-1957)

Fayol Theory (1841-1925)

Fayol was a French industrialist known as **Father of the management process school** concerned with management of production shops.

He studied the functions of managers and concluded that management is universal. He believed that:

1. All the managers regardless of the type of organization or their level in organization have essentially the same tasks such as planning, organizing, issuing orders, coordinating and controlling.
2. He derived general principles of administration from his observations:
   - He believed in the division of work.
   - He argued that specialization increases efficiency.
   - He recommended centralization through the use of scalar chain or levels of authority, responsibility accompanied by authority.
   - Unity of command and direction so that each employee receives orders from one superior.
   - He believed that although individual interests should be subordinated to agency's interest, workers should be allowed to think through and implement plans and should be adequately remunerated for their services.
   - Fayol encouraged development of group harmony through equal treatment and stability of tenure of personnel.
   - A firm believer of orderliness. He advocated that there is "a place for every thing and every thing in its place."
   - He also urged that management be taught in the colleges.

Max Webber Theory (1864-1920)

He is German psychologist. He earned the title of *father of organizational theory.* His emphasis was on rules instead of individuals and on competencies over favoritism. His conceptualization was on bureaucracy, a structure of authority that would facilitate the accomplishment of organizational objectives.

The three basis for authority:

1. Traditional authority, which is accepted because it seems things have always been that way such as the rule of a king in a monarchy.
2. Charisma, having a strong influential personality.
3. Rational legal authority which is considered rational in formal organizations because the person has demonstrated the knowledge, skills and ability to fulfill the position.

Webber recognized that if subordinates do not believe a person qualified for that position they may not accept that person's authority.

James Mooney Theory (1884-1957)

Mooney believed that management to be the technique of directing people and organization the technique of relating functions. Organization is managements responsibility.

Four universal principles of organization by Mooney:
1. Coordination and synchronization of activities for the accomplishment of a goal.
2. Functional effects, the performance of one's job description.
3. Scalar process organizes level of commands.
4. Arrange authority in to a higher archie.

Consequently people get their right to command from their position in the organization.

HUMAN RELATIONS THEORY

The human relations movement began in 1940s.
- Focused on the effect that the individuals have on the success or failure of an organization.
- Classic organization and management theory concentrated on the physical environment fail to analyze the human element.

Instead of concentrating on the organization's structure, managers encourage workers to develop their potentials and help them meet their needs for:
- Recognition
- Accomplishment
- Sense of belonging.

Two theorists who emphasized on human relations:
1. Follett –Mary Parker Follett (1868-1933)
2. Kurt Lewin (1890-1947)

Follett Theory (1868-1933)

- Follett stressed the importance of coordinating the psychological and sociological aspects of management in 1920s.
- She perceived the organization as a social system and management as a social process.
- She distinguished between power with others and power over others.
- Indicated that legitimate power is produced by a circular behavior where by superiors and subordinates mutually influence one another.
- The law of the situation dictates that a person does not take orders from an other person but from the situation.

Example
- Nurses work through lunch break during emergency or
- The faculty work after hours to organize conferences or

- Recruitment process or tutoring the students/counseling, etc.
- In factories extra production to meet the demands.

The disadvantage of this idea is that it is difficult for the workers to know the total situation.

- Follett advocated that the managers study the whole situation to achieve unity, because she believed that the control would be obtained through cooperation among all elements, people and materials.
- Her work was a link between the classic organization and human relations eras.

Lewin Theory (1890-1947)
- Lewin focused on the **Group Dynamics.**
- He maintained that groups have personalities of their own: composites of the members personalities.
- He showed that group forces can over come individual interests.

Example
An action can be taken according to the decision made by a group (majority) in a class, when different opinions given by other members of the class.

- Lewin focused on the Group Dynamics.
- He maintained that groups have personalities of their own: composites of the member's personalities.
- He showed that group forces can over come individual interests.

For example: A decision can be made in a class by taking majority from the group for taking any action. When there are different opinions by the other members of the class.

- Lewin advocated democratic supervision.
- His research indicated that.
- Democratic groups in which participants solve their own problems and have the opportunity to consult with the leader are most effective.
- Autocratic leadership on the other hand tends to promote hostility and aggression or apathy and decrease initiative.

BEHAVIORAL SCIENCE THEORY

Emphasis is on:
- Use of scientific procedures to study the psychological,
- Sociological, and
- Anthropological aspects of human behavior in organizations.

Behavioral Scientists Indicated
- The importance of maintaining a positive attitude toward people,
- Training managers,
- Fitting supervisory actions to the situation,
- Meeting employees needs,

- Promoting employees sense of achievement, and
- Obtaining commitment through participation in planning and decision making.

The two famous behavioral scientists are:
- Douglas McGregor (1932)
- Rensis Likerts (1903-1981)

McGregor's Theory

He developed the managerial implications of **Maslow's theory.**

He noted that one's style of management is dependent on one's philosophy of humans and categorized those assumptions as theory X and theory Y.

Theory X

- The manager's emphasis is on the goal of organization.
- The theory assumes that people dislike work and avoid it.

Consequences of theory X

- Workers must be directed,
- Controlled,
- Coerced, and
- Threatened
  So that organizational goals can be met.

According to theory X

- Most people want to be directed and to avoid responsibility because they have little ambition.
- They desire security.

Managers who accept the assumptions of theory X

- Will do the thinking and planning with little input from staff associates.
- They will delegate little, supervise closely.
- Motivate workers through fear and threats.
- Failing to make use of the workers potentials.

Theory Y

In theory Y, the emphasis is on the goal of individual. It is the manager's assumption that:
- People do not inherently dislike the work and that work can be a source of satisfaction.

- Workers have the self direction and self control necessary for meeting their objectives.
- Will respond to the rewards for the accomplishment of those goals.

Managers who believe in this Y' theory

- Will allow participation.
- They will delegate.
- Give general supervision than close supervision.
- Support job enlargement.
- Use positive incentives such as praise and recognition.

They believe that under favorable conditions: people seek responsibility and display imagination, unity and creativity.

According to theory Y' human potentials are only partially used.

Likert's Theory

His theory of management is based on his work at the University of Michigan's institute for social research.

He identified three variables in organizations.

1. The casual variable include leadership behavior.
2. The intervening variables are perceptions, attitudes, and motivations.
3. The end result variables are measures of profits, costs, and productivity.

Likert believes that the managers may act in ways harmful to the organization because they evaluate end results to the exclusion of intervening variables.

So, he developed a Likert scale questionnaire that includes measures of casual and intervening variables.

Factors Measured by Likert Scale

The scale measures several factors related to leadership behavior process:

- Motivation,
- Managerial influence,
- Communication,
- Decision making process,
- Goal setting, and
- Staff development.

Four types of management system according to Likert.

1. Exploitive—authoritative
2. Benevolent—authoritative
3. Consultative
4. Participative group

Effects of the Management Systems

1. Exploitive—authoritative
   - He associates the FIRST system with the least effective in performance.
   - Managers show less confidence in staff associates and ignore their ideas.
   - Consequently staff associates do not feel free to discuss their jobs with their managers.

2. Benevolent—authoritative
   - Staff associates ideas are sometimes sought, but they do not feel free to discuss their jobs with the manager.
   - Top and middle management are responsible for setting goals.
   - There is minimal communication. Mostly downward and received with suspicion.
   - Decisions are made at the top with some delegation.

3. Consultative system
   - The manager has substantial confidence in staff associates.
   - Their ideas are usually sought.
   - They feel free to discuss their jobs with the manager.
   - Goal setting is fairly general.
   - It has limited accuracy and accepted with some caution.
   - Broad policy is set at the top level.
   - There is decision making through out organization.
   - Control functions are delegated to lower levels where.
   - Reward and self guidance are used.
   - There is some resistance from informal groups in the organization.

4. Participative group

The fourth system is associated with the most effective performance. Managers have complete confidence in their staff associates. Their ideas are always sought, and they feel completely free to discuss their jobs with the manager. Goals are set at all levels. There is a great deal of communication – upward, downward, and lateral that is accurate and received with open mind.

Likert is strong believer of participative management and supportive relationships. His linking-pin concept is based on studies about the differences between good and poor managers as measured by their level of productivity. Good managers found to have more influence on their own managers than did poor managers. Their managerial abilities and procedures were better received by their staff associates. When middle managers have the opportunity for interaction with their manager, workers can have input and there is a chance for the individuals and the organizational goals to become similar.

Implications of Management Theories in Nursing

1. Taylor's theory can be implemented in nursing to study complexity of care and determine staffing needs and observe efficiency and nursing care.

2. Nurses can utilize Emerson's theory of early notion of the importance of objectives setting in an organization.
3. Nurses should be aware of the managerial tasks as defined by Fayol: Planning, Organizing, Directing, Coordinating and Controlling.
4. The theory of human relations of Follett and Lewin emphasis the importance for nurse managers to develop staff to their full potential and meeting their needs for recognition, accomplishment and sense of belonging.
5. Mc Gregon and Likert support the benefits of positive attitudes towards people, development of workers, satisfaction of their needs and commitment through participation.

The overall, study of the development of management theories, potential nurse leaders can define the role of management, develop leadership style, learn managerial techniques, and give an insight how to work with others to accomplish goals.

04 Leadership Theories

INTRODUCTION

There are many leadership theories and nurses can familiarize with the most common and adopt the most suitable for dealing with different situations.

Some of the common theories are discussed in this chapter (Fig. 4.1).

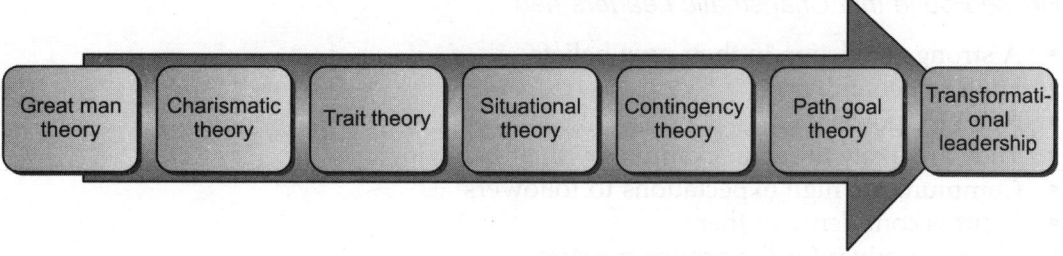

Fig. 4.1: Leadership theories

Great Man Theory

The great man theory argues that a few people are born with necessary characteristics to be great. Leaders are all round masters and display both instrumental and supportive leadership behavior.

Instrumental activities include planning, organizing, and controlling the activities of subordinates to accomplish the organizational goals. Obtaining and allocating resources such as people equipment materials funds and space are particularly important. Supportive leadership is socially oriented and allows for participation and consultation from subordinates for decisions that effect them.

People who use both instrumental and supportive leadership behaviors are considered as "Great Man" effective leaders in any situation.

Many find this theory **unattractive** because of its belief that the **leaders are born and not made,** which suggests that leadership cannot be developed.

Charismatic Theory

People may be Leaders because they are Charismatic

What constitutes charisma? Most agree that it is inspirational quality possessed by some people that make others feel better in their presence. The Charismatic leader inspires others by obtaining emotional commitment from followers and by arousing strong feelings of loyalty and enthusiasm. Under charismatic leader ship one may overcome obstacles not thought possible.

Yukl (1989), has reported findings from House's, Bass's, Conger and Kanungo's research about Charisma.

House's Research Findings

- Followers of charismatic leaders trust the leaders beliefs
- Have similar beliefs
- Exhibit affection for
- Obedience to
- And unquestioning acceptance of the leader
- Emotionally involved in;
- And believe they can contribute to mission.

House Found that Charismatic Leaders had

- A strong conviction in their own beliefs
- High self confidence
- Need for power
- They are likely to set an example by their behavior
- Communicate high expectations to followers
- Express confidence in them
- Arouse motives for the groups mission.

Conger and Kanungo's Research Findings

- They believe charisma is as attribution phenomena.
- It more likely attributed to leader advocates a vision discrepant from the status quo
- Emerges during a crisis
- Accurately assess the situation
- Communicates self confidence
- Uses personal power
- Makes self sacrifices
- Uses unconventional strategies.

Bass Proposed in his Research that

- Charismatic leaders perceive themselves as having supernatural purpose and destiny and that followers may idolize and worship them as spiritual figures or super humans.
- This blind obedience can lead to bad out comes such as group suicide.
- Transformational leaders use charisma for good.

Trait Theory

Until mid 1940s, the trait theory was the basis for most leadership research. Early work in this area maintained that traits are inherited, but later theories suggest that traits could be obtained through learning and experiences.

Researchers identified the leadership traits as:
- Energy
- Drive
- Enthusiasm
- Ambition
- Aggressiveness
- Decisiveness
- Self-assurance
- Self-confidence
- Friendliness
- Affection
- Honesty
- Fairness
- Loyalty
- Dependability
- Technical mastery
- Teaching skill

Later various researchers arrived at different conclusions and arrived at some common leadership traits (Fig. 4.2).

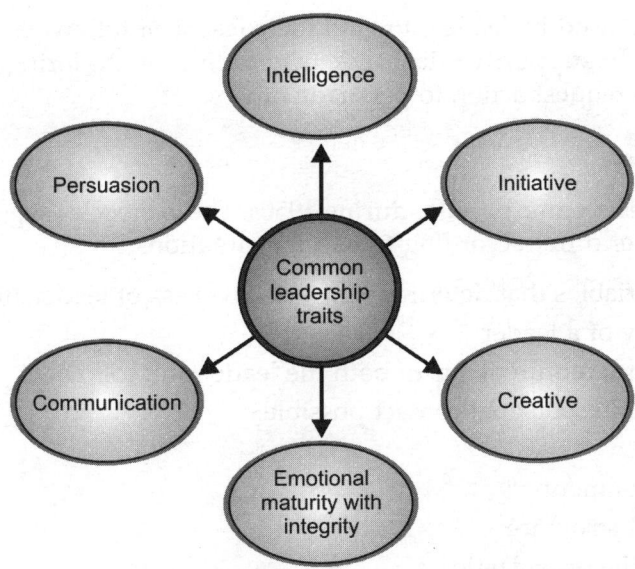

Fig. 4.2: Common leadership traits

Intelligence

Leaders need to be more intelligent than the group. However, a highly intelligent person may not find leadership responsibilities as challenging and may not be successful enough, and may prefer to work with abstract ideas and research.

Initiative

Leaders must be initiative and have the ability to perceive and start courses of action which are not considered by others.

Creative

Creativity is an asset. Having originality, the ability to think of new solutions to problems and ideas of new ways to be productive is helpful for a leader.

Emotional Maturity with Integrity

Emotional maturity is very much essential trait of a leader. Other traits are persistence, dependability, and objectivity. Mature leaders do what they say and are consistent in their actions which are referred to integrity.

Communication

Communication skills are important. The leader needs to understand others speak and write clearly.

Persuasion

Communication is used by leaders to gain the consent of followers. The leader make suggestions, supply supportive data, ask penetrating or exploring questions, make compromises and request action to persuade others.

Situational Theory

Situational theories became popular during 1950s. These theories suggest that the traits required of a leader differ according to varying situations.

Among the variables that determine the effectiveness of leadership such as:
- The personality of a leader
- The performance requirements of both the leader and followers
- The degree of interpersonal contact possible
- Time pressures
- Physical environment
- Organizational structure
- The nature of the organization
- The state of the organizations development
- The influence of the leader outside the group

A person may be a leader in one situation and a follower in other situations because the type leadership required depends on the situation.

Contingency Theory

Fred Fieldler introduced the contingency model of leadership in 1960s.

He argued that a leadership style will be effective or ineffective, dependent on the situation.

He identified three aspects of a situation that structures the leaders role.
1. Leader—member relations
2. Task structure
3. Position power

Leader member relations involve the amount of confidence and loyalty the followers have in their leader.

Task structure is high if it is easy to define and measure a task. The structure is low if it is difficult to define the task and to measure progress towards its completion. Fielder used four criteria to determine the degree of task structure.
1. Goal clarity and goal understood by the followers.
2. Extent to which a decision can be verified, know who is responsible for what.
3. Multiplicity of a goal paths, number of solutions.
4. Specificity of a solution: Number of correct answers.
   - Technical nursing, which focuses on procedures, may have numerous solutions involving human relations and value judgments may have numerous solutions with no specific correct answer and consequently have low task structure.
   - Position power refers to the authority inherent in a position. The power to use rewards and punishments and the organizations support of ones decisions.
   - Directors of nursing, managers, and sometimes patient care coordinators have high position, or be subjected to removal by peers or subordinators.
   - Elected committee chairpersons, team leaders and staff nurses usually have low position power.

Path Goal Theory

Robert J House derived path goal theory from expectancy theory.
- The expectancy theory argues that the people act as they do because they expect their behavior to produce satisfactory results.
- In the path-goal relationship, the leader facilitates task accomplishment by minimizing obstructions to the goals and by rewarding followers for completing their tasks.
- The leader helps the staff to assess the needs, explore alternatives.
- Helps them to make the most beneficial decisions.
- Rewards personnel for task achievements.
- Provides additional opportunities for satisfying goal accomplishments.

Transformational Leadership

Transformational leaders organize groups, around their personal goals and believe that others also motivated by personal goals.

Transformational leaders motivate others through:
- Values
- Vision
- Empowerment.

Bass (1985) has described transformational leaders in terms of charisma, inspirational leadership, individualized consideration and intellectual stimulation.

Bennis and Nanus (1985), indicate that:
- Leaders do the **right things**, where as managers do **things right**.
- Leaders focus on **effectiveness** and managers deal with **efficiency**.

The four strategies identified by Bennis and Nanus:
- *Attention through vision:* The leaders vision needs to be clear attractive and attainable.
- *Meaning through communication:* Open communications, honesty and consistency are important to be build trust.
- *Trust through positioning:* The leader's position must be clear because associates are more likely to be trusting when they know the leaders view of the organization.
- *Deployment of self.*

Hitt (1993) defines leadership as affecting people so that they will strive willingly towards group goals.

Hitt identified five types of knowledge needed by a leader (Fig. 4.3).

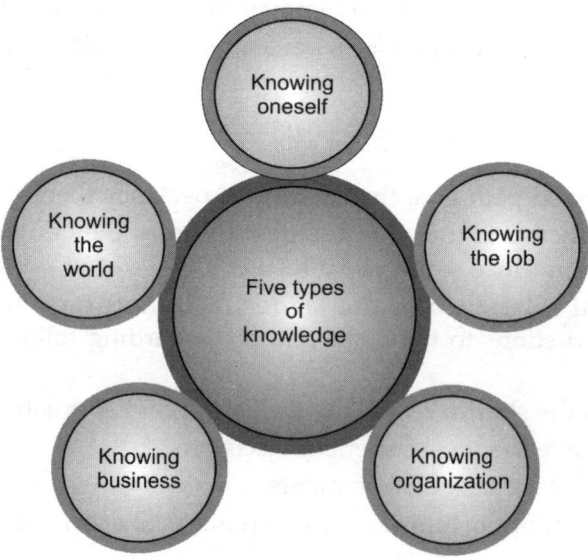

Fig. 4.3: Five types of knowledge

He also identified five core functions of a leader (Fig. 4.4).

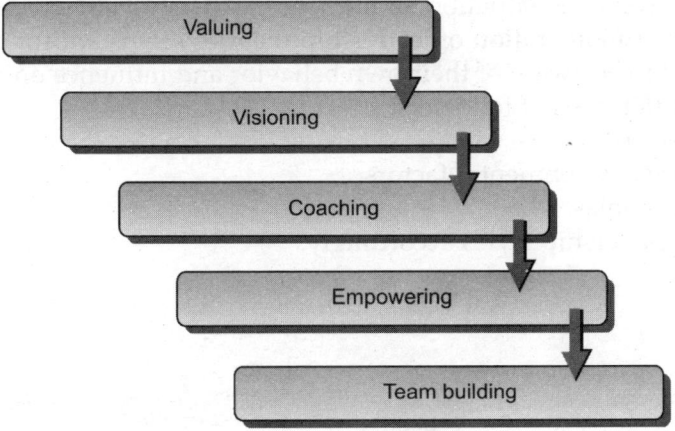

Fig. 4.4: Five core functions

He listed the six attributes essential for leadership as
- Identity
- Independence
- Authenticity
- Responsibility
- Courage
- Integrity

Integrative Leadership Model (ILM) (Fig. 4.5)

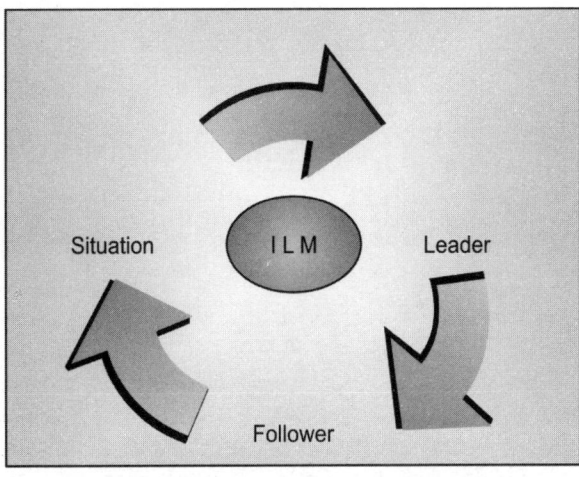

Fig. 4.5: Integrative leadership model (ILM)

From review of leadership theories, obiviously there is no one best leadership style. Leaders are rarely totally people or task oriented.
- Leaders, followers and situation all influence leadership effectiveness.
- Consequently an integration of leadership theories seems appropriate.
- Leaders need to be aware of their own behavior and influence on others.
- Individual differences of followers.
- Group characteristics.
- Task structure environmental factors.
- Situational variables.
- Adjust their leadership styles accordingly.

Example

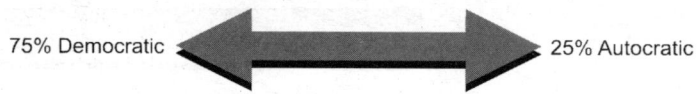

Finally leadership behavior needs to be adaptive

Unit III: Leadership Styles

05 Types of Leaders and Leadership Styles

OBJECTIVES

1. Define the concepts of leadership, style, and leadership styles.
2. Describe the three common leadership styles their advantages and disadvantages.
3. Discuss the effective leadership style and the qualities of a leader.
4. Analyze the structured situation provided for different type of leadership styles.

INTRODUCTION

Leadership does not mean dominating the subordinates. The leader's job is to get work done by other people, and make people willingly want to accomplish some thing. So effective leadership means effective and productive group performance.

DEFINITIONS

Leadership

Leadership is the process of influencing the thoughts and actions of other people (a person or a group) to attain the desired objectives.

Style

A style is a particular form of a behavior directly associated with an individual.
 Or, the way in which a leader uses interpersonal influences to achieve the objective of an organization. One should ask why the style of functioning of a leader need to be understood.

The reasons are:
- A style of leadership affects the health care delivery system.
- A style allows the nurse to interact more productively and more harmoniously to achieve personal and organizational goals.

Leadership Style

Leadership style is how a leader uses interpersonal influence to accomplish goals of an organization.

Types of Leadership Styles

There are four types:

Autocratic Style of Leadership

Autocratic leadership is described as:
- Authoritarian leadership
- Directive leadership and the leader is referred to as
- Extreme form of "Dictator"

Democratic Style of Leadership

A democratic leadership is described as:
- Participative or
- Consultative style of leadership.

Laissez-Faire Style of Leadership

Also known as:
- Permissive
- Free-rein
- Anarchic
- Ultraliberal style of leadership

Bureaucratic style of leadership—which amphasis rules and regulation.

AUTOCRATIC LEADERSHIP

The leader assumes complete control over the decisions and activities of the group. The authority for decision making is not delegated to persons in lower level positions (centralized organization).

Personality of the Leader

- Firm personality, insistent, self-assured, highly directive, dominating, with or without intention.
- Has high concern for work than for the people who perform the task.
- Uses the efforts of the workers to the best possible shows no regard to the interests of the employees.
- Sets rigid standards and methods of performance and expects the subordinates to obey the rules and follow the same.
- Makes all decisions by himself or herself related to the work and pass orders to the workers and expect them carry out the orders.
- There is minimal group participation or none from the workers.
- Thinks that what he or she plans and does is the best. May listen to them by not influenced by their suggestions.

- Has no trust or confidence in the subordinates in turn they fear and feel they have nothing much in common.
- Exercises power, manipulates the subordinates to act according to his goals plans and keeps at the center of attention.

Advantages and Disadvantages of Autocratic Leadership

Sl.No	Advantages	Disadvantages
1.	Efficient in times of crisis, easy to make decision by one person than by group and less time consuming.	Does not encourage the individuals growth and does not recognize the potentials, initiativeness and creates less cooperation among members.
2.	It is useful when there is only leader who is experienced having new and essential information while subordinates are in experienced and new.	The leader lacks supportive power that results in decisions made with consultation although he may be correct.
3.	It is useful when the workers are unsure of taking decision and expect the leader to tell them what to do.	Inhibits groups participation which results in lack of growth, less job satisfaction can lead to less commitment to the goals of organization.

DEMOCRATIC LEADERSHIP

It is also referred to participative, consultative style of leadership.
1. This style is characterized by a sense of 'equality' among leaders and followers.
    - The leader is people oriented
    - Focuses on the human aspects
    - Builds effective work group
    - Togetherness is emphasized
2. Open system of communication prevails.
    The group participate in work related decisions (sharing the thoughts in problem solving).
3. The interaction between the leader and the group is friendly and trusting.
    - The leader brings the subject to be discussed to the group
    - Consults
    - Decision of the majority is made and implemented by the entire group
    - Makes final decision after seeking input from the total group.
    - Therefore, the group feels they have important contribution to make, Freedom–ideas drawn, develop sense of responsibility for the good of the whole.
4. Leader works through people not by domination but by suggestions and persuasions
    - The leader motivates the workers to set their own goals, makes their own work plans and evaluates their own performance.
    - Informs the overall purpose and the progress of the organization.

5. Performance standards exist to provide guidelines and permit appraisal of workers, thus results in high productivity.

Advantages and Disadvantages of Democratic Leadership

Sl. No	Advantages	Disadvantage
1.	It permits and encourages all employees to practice decision making skills.	It takes more time for making the decisions by the group than by leader alone. However, the advantages over weigh the negative outcomes.
2.	It promotes personal involvement. Suggestions are welcomed. This results in greater commitment to work and enhanced job satisfaction	
3.	Decisions made by the group are more effective than by the leader alone. Members may have more information than the leader	

LAISSEZ–FAIRE LEADERSHIP

It is also referred to as Free-Rein, Anarchic, and Ultraliberal style of leadership. The leader gives up all power to the group.

Characteristic Features

1. This leadership encourages independent activity by the group members.
   - An outsider would not be able to identify the leader in such a group.
   - The leader exerts little or no influence on the group members.
   - There is lack of central direction, supervision, coordination and control.
2. Group members are free to set their own goals determine their own activities and allowed to do almost what they desire to do.
   A variety of goals may be set by every individual and it will be difficult to carry out to accomplish the task by the group easily.
3. This style may be chosen by the leader or it may evolve because:
   - The leader is too weak to exert any influence on the group.
   - Attempting to please every one to feel good.
   - Fails to function as an effective leader.
4. This style is effective in highly motivated professional groups. For example, research projects where independent thinking is rewarded or when the leader feels that the problem must be solved by the group alone.
5. This style is not useful in a highly structured health care delivery system or any institution.
6. The group where there is no appointed leader will fall in to this category.

Advantages and Disadvantages of Laissez-Faire Leadership Style

Sl.No	Advantages	Disadvantages
1.	In limited situations creativity may be encouraged for specific purposes. e.g. highly qualified people plan a new approach to a problem that need freedom of action	May lead to instability, disorganization, inefficiency, no unity of actions.
2.	To try new methods of actions	Neither the group nor any one in the group will feel to be responsible to solve the problems that may arise. The individual members will lose interest, initiative and desire for achievement.

BUREAUCRATIC STYLE OF LEADERSHIP

In this kind of leadership the leader functions only on lines with rules and regulations. The leader cannot be flexible and does not like to take any risk out of the rules.

Example

Defense leaders. They are strictly adhering to the rules and maintain the discipline of group.

The Effective Leadership Style

- No one functions always with a particular leadership style.
- No single style is appropriate for all situations.
- At times combination of styles may be most appropriate.

For example, a midway between authoritarian and democratic or between democratic and Laissez-Faire.

Comparison of Leadership Styles

Parameters	Authoritarian	Democratic	Laissez-Faire
Control over the group	Strong	Less	Little or none
Motivation	By coercion	Economic/Ego awards	By support
Direction	By command	Suggestion/guidance	Little, upward and downward
Decision making	Self	Participative	Dispersed
Status difference	I and U	We	The group
Criticism	Punitive	Constructive	None

The Factors which Influence the Leadership of a Nurse Manager

- The nature of work (ICU, regular unit)
- The characteristics of nursing staff (Knowledge, competencies, attitudes)
- The time available
- The importance of the results (quality of care)

The Qualities of a Leader (Fig. 5.1 A and B)

Managerial Abilities

- Plans, organizes, makes decisions effectively encourages cooperation and participation.
- Assists nurse/subordinates in solving the problems and provides consistent feedback.
- Provides rationale for difficult decisions.
- Assess abilities of the workers, guides them to develop new skills.
- Knows her/his job and does it well and has confidence in self and others.
- Welcomes different opinions and is more interested in giving than receiving.
- Provides the workers with adequate facilities.

Interpersonal Relationships

- Shows supportive and caring behavior towards subordinates.
- Is a good listener and sensitive to others needs.
- Guides and motivates to act and work together.
- Establishes relationships with all types of workers, and able to work with others harmoniously.

Temperament (Nature of a Person)

- Reliable, open, honest and sincere.
- Shows a sense of humor tactful, friendly and loyal.
- Calm and charismatic, modest neat and patient.
- Positive energetic, hard worker, happy and enthusiastic.
- Shows a balance between work and home life or personal life.

Credibility and Forward Thinking

- Acts as a role model and influences others.
- Acts as an activist, challenger, creative thinker, change agent, innovator, risk taker and courageous.
- Acts as a facilitator and solution seeker.

Managerical abilities
Interpersonal relationships
Temperament (nature of a person)
Credibility and forward thinking
Professionalism

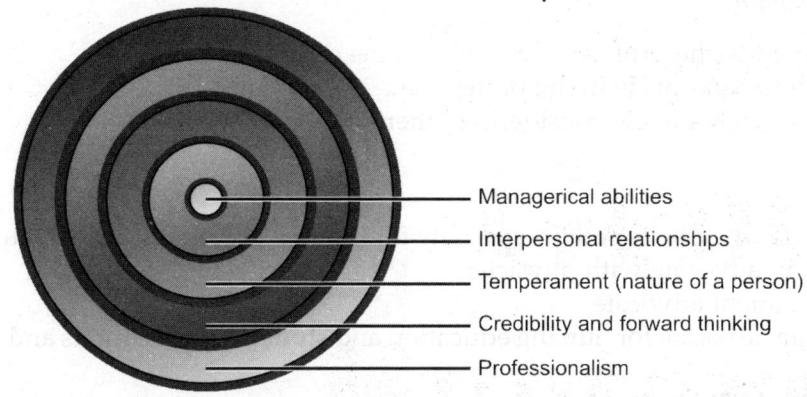

Fig. 5.1 A: Qualities of a leader

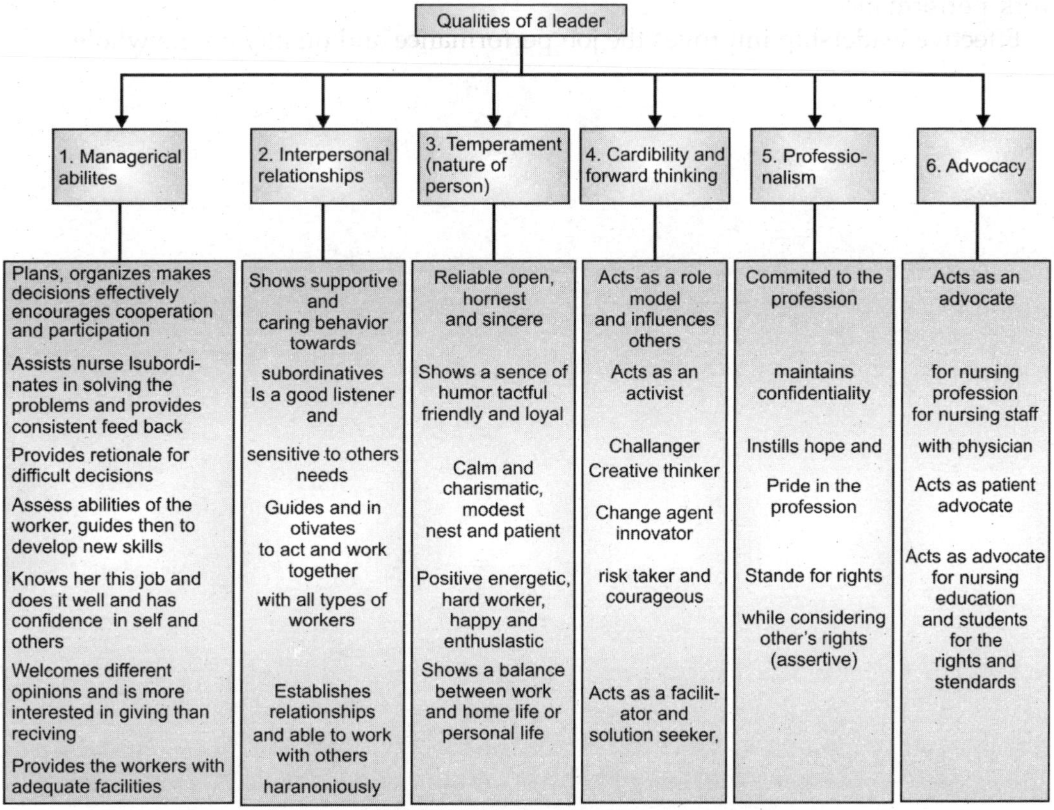

Qualities of a leader
1. Managerical abilites
2. Interpersonal relationships
3. Temperament (nature of person)
4. Cardibility and forward thinking
5. Professio-nalism
6. Advocacy
Plans, organizes makes decisions effectively encourages cooperation and participation
Assists nurse lsubordi-nates in solving the problems and provides consistent feed back
Provides retionale for difficult decisions
Assess abilities of the worker, guides then to develop new skills
Knows her this job and does it well and has confidence in self and others
Welcomes different opinions and is more interested in giving than reciving
Provides the workers with adequate facilities
Shows supportive and caring behavior towards
subordinatives Is a good listener and
sensitive to others needs
Guides and in otivates to act and work together
with all types of workers
Establishes relationships and able to work with others
haranoniously
Reliable open, hornest and sincere
Shows a sence of humor tactful friendly and loyal
Calm and charismatic, modest nest and patient
Positive energetic, hard worker, happy and enthuslastic
Shows a balance between work and home life or personal life
Acts as a role model and influences others
Acts as an activist
Challanger Creative thinker
Change agent innovator
risk taker and courageous
Acts as a facilit-ator and solution seeker,
Commited to the profession
maintains confidentiality
Instills hope and
Pride in the profession
Stande for rights
while considering other's rights (assertive)
Acts as an advocate
for nursing profession for nursing staff
with physician
Acts as patient advocate
Acts as advocate for nursing education and students for the rights and stendards

Fig. 5.1 B: Qualities and functions of a leader

Professionalism

- Committed to the profession and maintains confidentiality.
- Instills hope and pride in the profession.
- Stands for rights while considering other's rights (assertive).

Advocacy

- Acts as an advocate for others specially for nursing profession and for nursing staff.
- Acts as an advocate with physician.
- Acts as patient advocate.
- Acts as an advocate for nursing education and students for the rights and standards.

Implications to Nursing

Regardless of the style selected the nurse managers should be aware of the effect of the style adopted in the hospital, unit or educational institution, staff and on the level of work performance.

Effective leadership improves the job performance and quality on the whole.

06 Time Management

OBJECTIVES

1. Describe the concept and importance of time management.
2. Apply the principles of proper time management.
3. Discuss the importance of delegation and its impact on management.

INTRODUCTION

Time is constant that cannot be altered. The clock cannot be slowed down or speed up. Thus, time management is a misnomer. No one manages the time itself. But what is managed is simply self management.

The nurse manager has a limited time. Her work is typically a shift beginning and ending with activities and events. The eight hour shift may become ten hour work day. She or he is required to use time wisely and to work smarter not harder.

DEFINITION

Time management is the optimum use of the available time.

IMPORTANCE OF TIME

- To know how to use time wisely.
- To get more work done in less time.
- To conserve time and energy.

PRINCIPLES OF TIME MANAGEMENT

The nurse manager may start a plan for maximizing the use of managerial time by application of the following principles.

Selection of Staff

Section of well qualified staff is critical for time saving because they require less supervisory time for development and corrective action.

Appropriate use of staff through assessment of work and careful planning of the number and qualifications of personnel needed, and matching the staff member's interest and abilities to her / his job further reduce waste.

Also staffs that are adequately informed do not waste time wandering what to do. The availability of organization all charts and job descriptions save time to find out who is responsible to whom and for what, lines of authority, etc. Grouping similar activities in hospital unit also save time, i.e. medical unit, surgical unit, ICU.

Goal Setting

A critical component of time management is defining short- and long-term goals and time frames. Goals provide direction and vision for actions and a time line in which activities will be accomplished.

Five major questions about goals must be answered if the nurse manager is to manage time effectively.
1. What specific unit objectives are to be achieved?
2. What specific activities are necessary to achieve these objectives?
3. How much time is required for each activity?
4. Which activities can be planned and scheduled for current actions and which must be planned and scheduled sequentially?
5. Which activities can be delegated to staff?

Setting Priorities

Priorities should be established for the activities to be performed by the nurse manager. The nurse manager should take into account both the importance and urgency of activities.

Table 6.1 shows five types of activities with examples.

Table 6.1: Priority of activities

Sl.No	Category of time use	Examples
1.	Important and urgent	Replacing two call-offs and ensuring sufficient staffing for the upcoming shift
2.	Important and not urgent	Drafting an educational program for nurses on the changes in medical sciences and technology
3.	Urgent not important	Completing and submitting the "beds available" list for a disaster drill
4.	Busy work	Compiling new charts for future patient admissions
5.	Wasted time	Sitting by the phone waiting for return calls

Daily Planning and Scheduling

Once goals and priorities have been established, the nurse manager can concentrate on scheduling activities. A to-do list should be prepared each day. Either after work hours of the previous day or before starting the days works on the same day. The list is typically planned by work day or work week. As nurse managers combine many activities or responsibilities, a weekly to do list may be more effective. Flexibility must be a major concern in this plan. The nurse manager should leave sometime uncommitted to deal with the unexpected emergencies that are sure to happen. In building this plans each activity to be prioritized. The focus is not on the activities and events, but on the out comes that can be achieved in the time available.

A system to keep track of regularly scheduled meetings (staff meeting), regular events (annual or quarterly report due dates) and appointments is also necessary. This system should include both a calendar and files. The calendar might include information on the purpose of the meeting, who will be attending and the time and place. While a file might contain correspondence or reports related to the meeting. This file can be arranged by date so that it is readily available at the time needed.

Plan Strategies

Once the nurse manager has determined and worked out her / his goals, she or he plans the strategies for how to accomplish them. She decides what activities must be done what are low priority activities that can be eliminated and schedules activities.

As the nurse manger looks at her major responsibilities she balances the work load around tasks that have to be done at certain times, i.e. budget preparation, can regulate months, week at -a-glance, daily work sheets showing what work should be done each day, the time or a particular hour which may be useful.

Delegation

Delegation is the process by which responsibility, authority, and accountability for performing tasks (functions, activities, and decisions) are assigned to individuals. A variety of activities may be delegated by the nurse manager.

Delegation involves assign tasks, determining expected results, and granting authority to the individual to accomplish these tasks. It means conveying rights and obligations to a subordinate.

Concepts related to delegation include responsibility, accountability and authority.
a. Responsibility means that the subordinate has an obligation to carry out the activities needed to accomplish the assigned task.
b. Accountability is being held answerable for the results.
c. Authority is the power to make final decisions and to command. The nurse manager may delegate tasks to another individual, but she and the delegate are both answerable for the results or lack of them.

Personal Organization and Self-discipline

The nurse manager is involved in many activities, situations, and events in relation to time available. The nurse manager must be personally well-organized and possess self discipline in order to be effective, i.e. to focus in one task at a time, making sure to start with a high priority task.

Improve Reading and Memory

- Learning speed reading can help in overcoming reading problems and inability to concentrate.
- Listening and memory techniques also save time. When listening for understanding the nurse manger should be attentive, delaying judgment, maintain eye contact and using attentive body language.
- Distractions affect concentration and should be reduced.
- To stimulate memory follow some of the simple techniques like Verbal techniques (repeating, clarifying), mental techniques (focusing and linking), physical techniques (notes taking, filing).

Transition Time

Much time is spent in transition or waiting, i.e. for meeting to start or to talk to some one, etc. This time can be used effectively by bringing materials to read or work.

Use Telephone Calls

- Use telephone instead of office visits or correspondence save time.
- Secretaries can screen calls so that other activities are not interrupted and may be able to handle them.
- A call-back system can be used or cordless phone allows one to move around and work. Nowadays mobile phones are making the life very much easy and comfortably have an easy access to people across the Globe.

Schedule Office Visits

The secretary can schedule appointment for the appropriate and inform the nurse manager of the purpose of the meeting so that she/he can be adequately prepared. Closing office door is helpful to complete the talk without interruption.

Say 'No'

Most people find it difficult to say "no" to a responsible request from a coworker. However, learning how to say no firmly and tactfully and with a pleasant facial expression saves time. Under the following conditions, a nurse manager should refuse to undertake responsibilities that are not her/his required job duties.

Such as:
1. When the activity will not serve the managers own professional goals.
2. When the activity requires time and abilities that the manager does not have.
3. When the activity holds no interest for the manager.
4. When undertaking the activity will prevent the manager's involvement in more attractive or more rewarding activity.

Use Meetings Effectively

- Meetings should start on time.
- Stating the purpose of the meeting and following the agenda are the nurse manager's responsibility.
- She or he should start with high priority items.
- Control interruptions.
- Restate conclusions.
- Make assignments and dead lines clear and ends the meeting on time.
- Minutes are circulated preferably within a day after the meeting. This allows staff to be informed without having to attend the meeting unless their input is needed. Minutes also remind staff of their assigned tasks.

Schedule Paper Work

Nurse managers spend considerable time in writing and reading and they are required to cope with increasing unit paperwork.

Some measures can be followed by the nurse manager.

- Plan schedule time for paper work, i.e. time for recording, time to answer mails.
- Sort paper work for effective processing, i.e. system of filing.
- Share paper work responsibilities with the staff, i.e. teaching staff.
- Write the mails effectively to avoid rewritings.
- Analyze paper work frequently, i.e. standard forms, reports and use color coding, etc.
- Do not be paper shuffler, i.e. do not keep papers on desk, handle them for action.

Time Analysis

The nurse manger analyzes the duties to be performed as specified in the job description, *and conducts a survey of the actual time spent on various activities to determine:*

- How time is used?
- Patterns of time used?
- Which activities are essential?
- Which can be delegated or eliminated?
- How to reduce time wasters?

Evaluation

The nurse manager should at least make a weekly assessment of how effectively time has been used. A good time to complete this review is while identifying priorities for the next week.

Respecting Time

Finally, the key to use time management is to respect one's own time as well as that of others, i.e. using the above measures regarding time management communicate to those who interact with the nurse manager that respect for time is demanded.

The nurse manager in managing the nursing unit should continually ask how can I use the time most effectively?

In general, good management in a nursing unit conserves time and energy.
Key terms of time management
Is
The optimum use of the available time.

EXERCISE

Identify the leadership qualities and styles necessary to carry out the priority tasks in the most efficient way.

Guidelines

- The teacher may divide the group in to small sub-groups.
- Ask each group to list **five** best qualities they would like to see in their leader and give reasons —why?
- Specify the tasks carried out by the following nursing personnel on a daily basis with priority.
  1. Principal
  2. Nursing superintendent
  3. Ward nurse or In-charge
  4. Lecturer
  5. Tutor

Present the group work to the class.

07 Communication and Critical Thinking in Management

OBJECTIVES

- Discuss the concept and levels of communication.
- Describe the communication model and its importance.
- Discuss the channels of managerial communication.
- Analyze the role of critical thinking in communication.

INTRODUCTION

Nurse managers are required to be aware of the techniques that can help them ensure effective management of educational / service unit.

Communication is one of the most important activities in the nursing management (Fig. 7.1). In fact communication is a managerial function. It is the foundation upon which the manager achieves organizational objectives.

Communication in a job is every one's job in the organization. Therefore, knowledge of communication and critical thinking is essential if effective working relationships are to be developed and maintained.

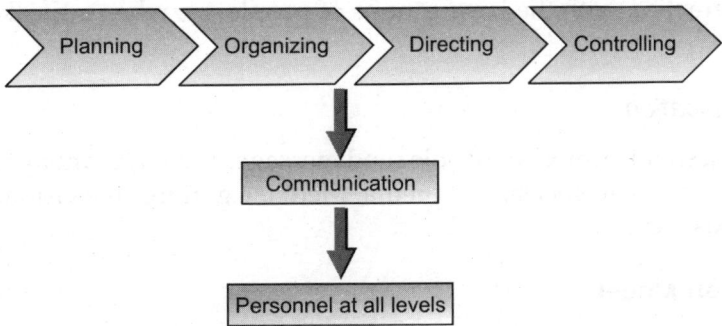

Fig. 7.1: Communication in management process

DEFINITION

Communication is a process in which a message is transferred from one person (sender) to other person (receiver) through a suitable media and the intended message is received and understood by the receiver.

Levels of Communication

Communication takes place in the management at various levels every day with various levels of people every day.

Intrapersonal Communication

It occurs when a person communicates with him self, i.e. when the individual looks out side and sees that it is very hot to go out during mid-afternoon and thinks to carry an umbrella with him.

Interpersonal Communication

Is referred to when a communication takes place between two people either face-to-face, or telephone, or small groups, etc.

Small Group Communication

It is referred to when a communication occurs between three or more people interacting with each other.

Organizational Communication

This refers to the communication takes place between members of an organization during the performance of organizational tasks, i.e. hospital, or educational institution, etc.

Public Communication

It involves interaction with the large groups of people, i.e. when a speaker address an audience.

Mass Communication

It occurs when a small number of people send messages to a large, anonymous audience through the use of some specialized media. Media, e.g. films, television, radio, newspapers and books, etc.

Communication Model

The goal of effective communication is understanding, not agreement or persuasion. Understanding builds productive relationships and opens the door for agreement or persuasion, e.g. the first line nurse manager can send a message to the blood bank for a unit of packed cells, but if it is not received or understood by some one which means no communication has occurred.

OR

If an HOD has given the message to the class representative regarding the change of time table for the class and no student turns up as per the change suggested then it means the message is not understood clearly by the student representative or the message is not reached respective class.

Effective communication is important for effective functioning.

An effective communication model consists of six steps for effective communication process.

1. The message
2. Encoding
3. Transmitting
4. Decoding action
5. Continuous feedback

Senders must have something to say before they send a message and that must be goal directed.

Message is the content of intended communication.

- **The Sender:** The sender chooses affect, concept idea or feeling to communicate. This is the content of communication. It is the basis of a message, e.g. the first line manager (sender) communicates information about patients, without a reason or goal, and there is no need for her/him to begin the communication process.
- **Encoding** is translating the message in to verbal (words) or non-verbal means (Expressions and gestures) that will communicate the intended message to the receiver.
- **Transmitting** is the channel used to communicate the message. The message may be in any form that can be understood by receiver's senses.

  For example, speech can be heard; can be written word (read) electronic media (slides, projectors TV) gestures facial expressions (seen or felt), A touch (comfort).

  Nonverbal messages area more honest than verbal messages.
- **Decoding:** The receiver perceives and interprets or decodes the sender's message into information that has meaning. The intended meaning will be communicated when the receiver and the sender have common experience, in other words, the effectiveness of the communication process depends on commonality of experiences.

  Therefore, one must speak the language of the other when people with different experience communicate.
- **Action:** It is the behavior adopted by the receiver as a result of the message sent received and perceived. It is the process of doing or performing something.
- **Communication** is not successful until the message received has been understood and acted upon appropriately.
- **Feedback:** It is a continuous two way process in which senders(s) receiver(s) exchange information and clarify meaning if the message sent. The communication process is not complete until feedback occurs. The greater the feedback, the more effective the so,

  Communication means that the instructions given (sender) have been understood, accepted and carried out (receiver).

Communication Model (Fig. 7.2)

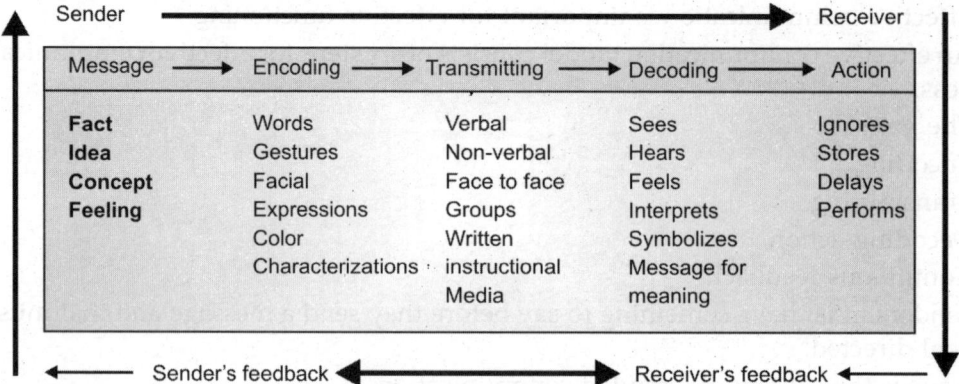

Fig. 7.2: Process of communication

Importance of Communication

a. It is the means through which nursing management achieves organizational goals.
b. Nursing managers in carrying out their management functions, spend most of the time communicating, i.e. with the nursing personnel, physicians, staff in supportive services, patients/ clients, etc.
c. Communication motivates staff members, i.e. sharing information of mutual interests, explaining plans, etc.
d. Communication leads to influence and power, i.e. the first line nurse manager can exert influence to institute measures to improve quality patient care.
e. It reduces anxiety, misunderstanding prejudices and enhances better interpersonal relationships.

Channels of Managerial Communications

There are four levels of managerial communications.

Downward Communication (Fig. 7.3)

This is the traditional and most commonly used communication, where the management gives orders to the subordinates at the bottom level to carry out the orders as per the organizational hierarchy.

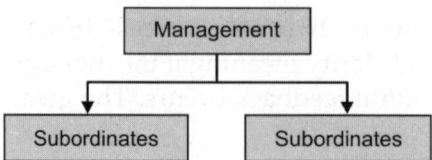

Fig. 7.3: Downward communication

Common means of downward communications are:
All the oral and written communications which are carried out from the top management to the employees by various means in order that the employees carry out their duties in the organization in achieving its Goals.

For example, Individual and group instructions, handbooks, operating manuals, job descriptions, performance appraisal, interviews, employee counseling, a loudspeaker, letters, memos, posters, bulletin boards, annual reports, etc.

Disadvantage: Downward communication contributes to greater dissatisfaction than upward communication regardless of the quality of message.

Upward Communication (Fig. 7.4)

Newer management technique encourages delegation of authority and more personnel involvement in decision making, thus creating a need for accurate upward communication.

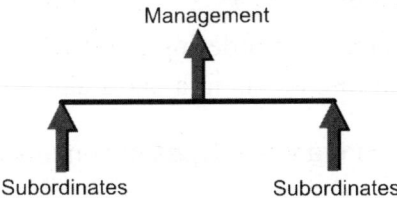

Fig. 7.4: Upward communication

Upward communication in the management travels from staff, lower and middle management personnel and continuous up to the organizational hierarchy. It provides a means for motivating satisfying personnel by encouraging employees input.

Common means for upward communication include; Face-to-face discussion, open-door policies, staff meetings, task forces, written reports, self-assessment appraisals, attitude surveys on job satisfaction, suggestion boxes. These encourage participative democratic management in the organization.

Lateral Communication (Fig. 7.5)

Lateral or horizontal communication is referred to the communication which takes place between the departments or personnel on the same level of the hierarchy.

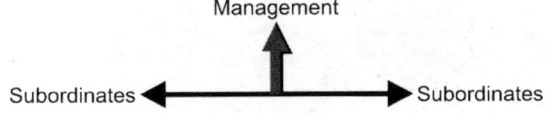

Fig. 7.5: Lateral communication

The need for lateral communication increases as interdependence increases.

Common means are; committees, conferences and meetings with the purpose of sharing information and solving the problems.

Diagonal Communication (Fig. 7.6)

Diagonal communication occurs between two individuals or departments that are not on the same level of the hierarchy.

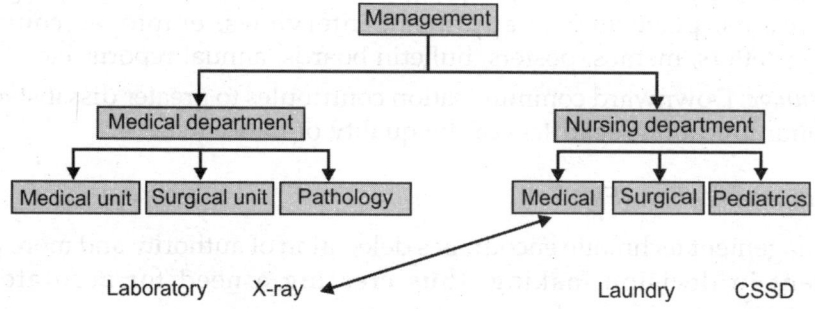

Fig. 7.6: Diagonal communication

Common means are: Unit in-charge ordering diet for the patient, X-ray department informs appointments given to patients in a particular unit, etc.

Types of Communication: There are two types of communication.

1. **Verbal communication:** Using spoken language or written language.
2. **Non-verbal communication:** Using gestures, postures, facial expressions, body movements, clothing grooming, etc. Everything communicates to other person what we are in the organization and depicts the image of a manager and his/her personality.

Critical Thinking in Communication (Fig. 7.7)

Communication as an essential skill to nurse managers, they need to think and be conscious of different angles in their communication in order to perform their roles as managers effectively.

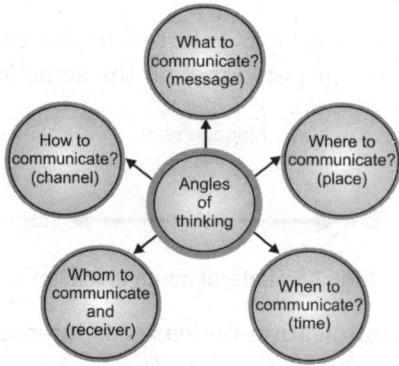

Fig. 7.7: Angles of thinking

Once, the managers understand these angles and can easily overcome the barriers which they come across in their daily routines.

The potential barriers to effective communication include:
- Time pressure
- Environmental interference
- Lack of information
- Complexity in the channel of communication, etc.

Nurses in what ever level they function, should attempt to over come by:
a. Establishing excellence in verbal, and non-verbal, and written communication.
b. Developing active listening skills.
c. Encouraging feedback from the receiver to help and eliminate discarded communication.
d. Focusing more on lateral communication than a downward communication.
e. Recognizing the importance of informal lines of communication.

Communication needs critical thinking and analysis of the situations in the management.

08 Group Dynamics

OBJECTIVES

1. Differentiate between group process and group dynamic.
2. Describe the four phases of group development.
3. Analyze the importance of establishing group norms in group dynamic.
4. Explain the reasons why nurses should form groups in their working environment.

INTRODUCTION

A group is an association of two or more people in an interdependent relationship with shared purposes.

What is known as group process?

"A group process is known as *when* a group works together to achieve certain goal" in any setting.

What is group dynamics?

Group dynamics is referred to as when there is a specific communication and interaction between the group members.

Types of Groups

There are two types:

1. *The formal work groups:* This is also known as *Task force*. It has clearly defined task to meet the organizational goals. In health care this means providing quality care according to clearly defined standards.
2. *The informal or social group:* The purposes of this group is to meet for companionship and socialization, e.g. clubs.
   The member's main goal is to reinforce friendship and minimize work related stress.

Phases of Group Dynamics

There are four distinguished phases (Fig. 8.1).

Phase 1: *Dependent phase:* This is a forming phase.
- Members are insecure and anxious
- Need each others support

Phase 2: *Independent phase:* Members start to be aware of the rules, roles and norms.
- Start to feel the group connections.
- But may feel intense and conflicts may arise.
- Conscious of themselves.

Phase 3: *Interdependent phase:* This known as *forming* and *performing phase.*
- Members have strong identity
- Trust one another
- Feel responsible for the task.
- Goal is defined, rules and roles are clearly defined and established and accepted.
- They perceive group goals are more important over individual interest.

Phase 4: *Termination phase:* This is known as adjourning phase or last phase.
- The group task has been completed and
- Members prepare to leave the group.

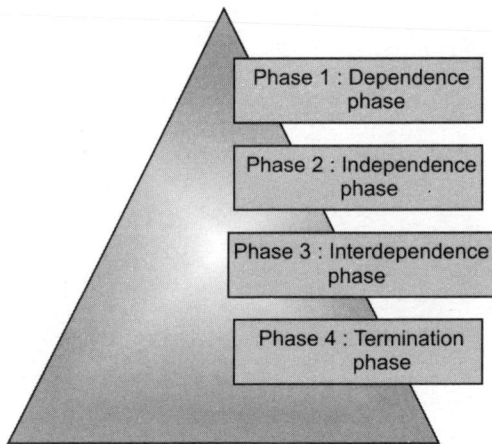

Fig. 8.1: Four phases of group dynamics

Group Size

- The size of the group is an important factor. If size increases the complexity of the dynamic increases.
- Ideal size of the work group should be 6-8 members.
- Small groups promote satisfaction and effective group process.

How are the groups guided?

They are guided by group norms and values.
These are the standards which shape *the behavior, attitude and perceptions* of members within the group.

Group Dynamics and its Application to Nursing

- To understand its process which would help the nurse to be more effective member of the group?
- The nurse leader is responsible for coordinating the group work to accomplish its goals of the unit.
- It helps the nurse leader to take appropriate actions effectively.
- Solve the problem encountered in the group.

Part B: Management of Nursing Practice in Health Care Agencies

Unit IV: Planning

09 Planning Process

OBJECTIVES

- Explain the definition, concept, purposes and activities of planning.
- Describe the types of planning.
- Discuss the elements of planning.
- Describe the kinds of data to be collected and analyzed for planning.
- Specify the points which leads to successful organizational planning.
- Identify the practical aspects of actions in day-to-day planning.

INTRODUCTION

Planning is the first step in the management process and every manager is expected to understand the essence of planning in true sense in order to be successful in their managerial role.

Planning is art of *thinking a head of time* or well in advance with regard to what needs to be done in an organized way to minimize the confusions in carrying out future actions.

THE PLANNING PROCESS

The process of planning needs thinking on the series of actions to be taken and directs attention to the objectives of an organization. It provides a manager with the means of control and encourages the best use of resources. Planning precedes all other management functions.

Planning requires vision, creativity, flexibility and energy in the planner. The nurse manager needs to be familiar with the decision making process and tools. So that she can identify the purpose of the institution, state the philosophy and policies, define goals and objectives, prepare budgets to implement plans, and effectively manage her/his time and that of the organization.

DEFINITION

Planning

It may be defined as determining what is to be achieved. It can also be defined as having a specific aim or purpose and mapping out a program or method beforehand and for accomplishment of goals.

Planning Process

It is a systematic process and requires knowledgeable activity based on managerial theory.

Purpose of Planning

- Planning leads to success in achieving goals and objectives
- It gives meaning to work
- Provides means to the effective use of available resources such as personnel and facilities in the organization
- Helps to cope with situational crisis
- It is cost effective and needed for effective control
- Planning is based on the past and future, thus helping to reduce the element of change and to discover need for change.

Activities of Planning

- Assessment; collect relevant data, classify, analyze, interpret and translate the data as a meaningful whole
- Identification of needs
- Priority setting
- Development of strategies
- Management of objectives: Formulation of policies, rules, regulations, methods and procedures.

Nursing is a clinical practice discipline providing service to human beings. So nurse managers need to plan in order to nurture the nurse practitioners who provide the service. Nurse educators in the educational institutions the novice teachers to be efficient in preparing the student nurses with right kind of values and knowledge.

The major function of planning includes both strategic and tactical planning:

Strategic Planning

This also is referred to as long-term planning which involves determining the direction in which an organization should be headed. Long-term plans are related to 3-5 years of range to achieve the management objectives.

Tactical Planning

It is referred to short-term planning. They are related to fiscal year (Yearly planning) which involves;
a. Allocating resources that enable an organization to reach strategic objectives.
b. Plans are mechanisms for guiding organizational efforts.
c. It is a continuous process, moves from setting mission to setting operational objectives.
d. Plans support evaluation.

Strategic Planning

Definition

It is a continuous systematic process of making risk-taking decisions to-day with the greatest possible knowledge of their effects on the future. Organizing efforts necessary to carryout these decisions and evaluating results of these decisions and evaluating results of these decisions against expected outcome through reliable feedback mechanisms.

Strategic planning in nursing is concerned with:
What is role of nursing division in strategic planning?
- To improve allocation of resources, time and money and to manage the division of nursing for performance of 3-20 years of time.
- Participants in planning should include from the TOP nursing management including clinical nursing personnel.

How can strategic planning be useful in improving nursing management?
- To provide accountability and monitoring of performance, tie merit to performance.
- To set up more formal planning programs and require divisional and unit planning.
- To integrate plans with operational and financial plans.
- To think more and concentrate on strategic issues.
- To improve knowledge of, and training in strategic planning.
- To increase top management involvement and commitment.
- To improve focus on completion, market segment, and external factors.
- To improve communication from top administration and nursing management.
- To allow better execution of plans.
- To use more realism and less rationalizing and vacillating.
- To improve the development of nursing management strategies.
- To improve the development and communication of nursing management goals.
- To put less emphasis on raw numbers.

Kinds of data that must be collected and analyzed for planning:
- Daily average patient census
- Average length of stay
- Bed capacity and percent of occupancy
- Number of births/operations
- Trends in patient's population; age, diagnosis. Acuity, physical dependency, etc.
- Trends in technology; diagnostic/ therapeutic
- Environmental; Nursing personnel, education, accreditation,
- Trends in health care system
- Trends in nursing; opportunities of nursing profession'.

Elements in planning:
- Written statements of mission/purpose
- Philosophy
- Objectives
- Detailed management plans, or strategies, policies and procedures.

Day-to-day planning activities of the nurse manager:
A practical day-to-day planning by the nurse manager has a great value in managing her unit.
- At the beginning of each day, make a list of actions to be completed for the day. Cross off the actions as they are accomplished or at the end of the day.
- Carry over actions which are not completed to the next day either do them first or decide whether those need to be done at all.
- Plan a head for the meetings. Distribute agenda in advance.
- For organizational meetings, send the nursing items to be included in the agenda and prepare for the meeting.
- Identify developing problems and put them in appropriate portion of the management plans.
- Review the plan on a scheduled basis with the key managers so that each knows the personal responsibilities for the activities.
- Review the appropriate portions of the development plan with the subordinate managers when they are counseled. Department, unit or clinic plans be reviewed at the same time.
- Seven day plan for the discussion of ideas from professional journals to integrate research results in to practice.
- Plan for educational programs for student educational experiences in the division of nursing.
- Plan for evaluation of clinical administrative practices to decide whether the objectives are achieved.

10 Decision Making and Problem Solving

OBJECTIVES
1. Discuss the concepts of decision making and problem solving approach.
2. Relate the process of decision making with the problem solving approach.
3. Explain the purposes of decision making.
4. Identify and apply the steps in the decision making process and problem solving in a systematic and comprehensive manner.

INTRODUCTION

The competent management of a leader depends on the sound judgments he/she makes in solving the problems and day-to-day issues in the organization.

Decision making is a necessary competent of a leadership, power, influence, authority and delegation (John 1993). Decisions call for judgments which result either in the organizations running effectively and efficiently or inefficient management and poor patient care. Decision making calls for systematic process in which a manager chooses among the alternatives, come to a conclusion and select an action.

Decision making versus problem solving are commonly used together. Sometimes these terms are associated with the nursing process. Problem solving and nursing process are very much similar.

SIMILARITIES

Sl. No	Nursing process	Problem solving
1.	Assessing	Identification of problem
2.	Analyzing	Gather information
3.	Diagnosing	Analyze information
4.	Planning interventions	Establish goal and seek alternatives
5.	Implementation	Implement strategy
6.	Evaluating	Evaluate out come

The most effective decision making involves a systematic process that is comprehensive and which focuses on predetermine outcomes.

ADVANTAGES

A comprehensive and systematic approach in decision making has many advantages:
1. It is characterized by order and direction that enables managers to determine where they are.

2. Provide a framework for data gathering which is relevant to the decision.
3. Allows application of previous knowledge and experiences that minimize errors and improve quality of patient care and work of an organization.
4. Increase manager's confidence and ability to make sound decisions.

STEPS IN DECISION MAKING PROCESS

There are six important steps which are most commonly used to make appropriate decisions.

Steps	Actions to be taken
Step I	• Identify and define the area of concern • It is critical before taking any step to take a decision • To be clear about the problem or concern you are addressing.
Step II	• Gather and analyze information. • Try together all the necessary information about the problem or concern in order to accurately understanding the situation. • Decision make without adequate information would not produce on appropriate result. • In gathering information, the manager depends on good communication and assessment skills. Once you gather enough information, you will than analyze and interpret the data. This is an essential steps where information is critically analyzed and dealt with.
Step III	• Establish goals. • This is an essential step prior to proper planning and taking a decisive action. • At this stage a manager should consider what he needs to accomplish and when. In addition one should draw specific criteria to measure the anticipate outcome.
Step IV	• Seek alternatives. • There are frequently several approaches to any given problem or concern. • The more strategies you generate, the more likely you are to identify an effective action. Then, from the alternatives you will determine the appropriate action to be taken. • In this phase of the decision making process, you will use your knowledge, experiences and review the ability of your team members. • Your alternative choice should also be taken into consideration its consequences. • Then choose the alternative which will most likely achieve the desired outcome.
Step V	• Implement the selected strategy. • Once the strategy has been selected, it follows logically that it will be implemented. In this phase the managers should decide who will implement the decision. • It is necessary to know that the manager remains responsible and accountable for the outcome. • Because the manager is still responsible and accountable for the outcome, he will have to maintain amount of control over the implementation. • A sound communication skill and a clear guideline is necessary to achieve the expected outcome.
Step VI	• Evaluate outcomes. • This is a final step of the decision making process. • In this phase, the manager will compare the actual outcomes from the desired outcome. • If the decision was effective, then the actual matches the desired outcomes. • If not effective, then the situation remains the same or perhaps worse than the original status.

You may wish to evaluate other factors such as efforts and time and the impact on staff or organization and ultimately the cost involved. If you were not satisfied, you will want to consider other alternatives to similar concerns in the future.

If your decision was ineffective you will need to review the steps again.
Take into consideration the following.
1. Problems/concerns were not correctly identified.
2. Assessment was not complete or properly analyzed.
3. Goals were unrealistic.
4. Decision taken without considering other possible alternatives and consequences.
5. The strategy chosen was incorrectly implemented due to lack of specific guidelines.
6. Evaluation of responses was incomplete or situation changed rapidly.

11
Budgeting

OBJECTIVES
1. Define the concept of fiscal planning, budgeting, and cost.
2. Identify the steps in budgeting process.

INTRODUCTION

Health economics has gained a lot to do in the management of health care agencies and in provision of effective and economical health care to individuals, families and community and country as a whole.

It is the responsibility of every country to look in to the sources of income over expenditure on various aspects of health which include education, infrastructure and organization of health care services.

- Fiscal planning is concerned with budget planning.
- It is vital because the ultimate survival of an organization largely depends on how proficiently funds are acquired and utilized.
- Fiscal planning monitors financial health of an organization.
- Fiscal planning must be proactive, flexible, and clearly stated in measurable terms.

Fiscal Planning Includes:

- Short-term planning,
- Long-term planning,
- Involves as many people as feasible.

Budgeting and Nursing

The economic welfare of a health agency depends on the effective budgeting for nursing department operations, because The nursing budget represents one-third of total operating budget.

What do the nurse managers need to know about budgeting?
1. Different types of expenditure.
2. Budgeting process.
3. Cost involved in carrying out different nursing activities.

Budgeting

- It is the allocation of scarce resources on the basis of *forecasted* needs for the *proposed* activities over a specified period of time.

- It is a *numerical* expression of an agency's *expected out come* and planned *expenditure*, and it is a tool for planning monitoring and controlling the income and expenditure.

Purpose of Budgeting

Primary Purpose

To ensure the most effective use of scarce financial and non-financial resources.

Other Purposes

- Coordinating efforts of various departments.
- Establishing a frame of reference for the managerial decision-making.
- Providing a criterion for evaluating managerial performance.

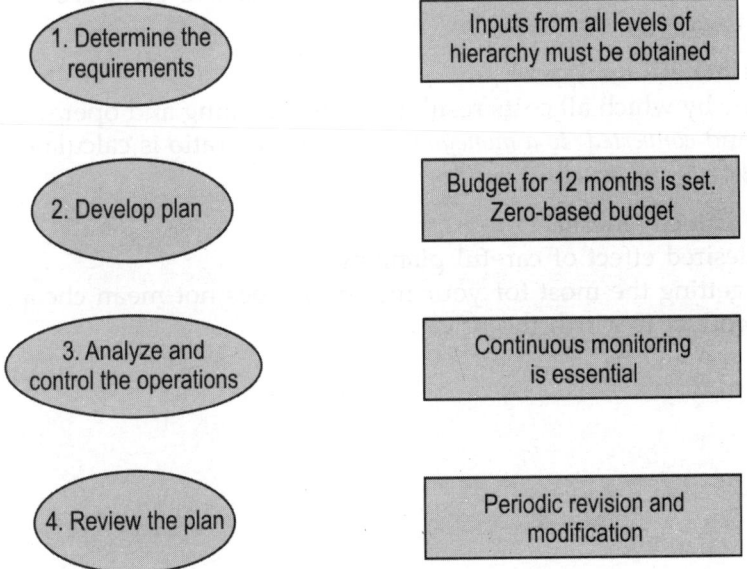

Fig. 11.1: Steps in budgeting process: (Douglas and Bavis 1983)

Types of Expenditure

Budgeting: It is management function of providing exployees with whatever is needed to carry out task.

Personnel Budget

It is the largest budget expenditure, e.g. salaries, productive time, etc.

Operating Budget

It includes daily expenditure, e.g. water, repairs, etc.

Capital Budget

It is for long life, e.g. purchase of buildings, major equipment.

Costs

It is the expenditure required to achieve a desired objective.
1. Direct costs include wages paid to the employees involved in productive work.
2. Indirect costs refers, all labor cost which is not included in direct costs.
3. **Cost accounting:** It is support service that provides managers with inf. for planning and evaluation.
4. **Cost reduction:** It is an adjustment function used to conserve scarce resources and ensure agency survival.

What is cost benefit analyses?

It is a procedure by which all costs resulting from installing and operating a system are determined and *converted to a money amount,* and the ratio is calculated to reflect the *relationship of costs and benefits.*

What is cost Effectiveness?

- It is the desired effect of careful planning.
- It means getting the most for your money. It does not mean cheap.
- But the product is worth the price.

Unit V: Organizing

12. Systems Theory and Systems Analysis

OBJECTIVES

1. Define systems theory and systems analysis.
2. Describe classic system elements.
3. Identifies the basic principles underlying the systems approach to nursing management.
4. Aware of advantages and disadvantages of systems approach.
5. Discuss the significance of systems theory to nurse manager.

INTRODUCTION

- Once the plans are made, the mission, philosophy.
- Objectives are established.
  The resources are organized to sustain philosophy and to accomplish the mission and objectives.

TYPES OF SYSTEMS

Closed/Open System

- Closed systems are self-contained.
- Open systems recognizes the interaction of the system with its environment.

Systems Theory

In a system there are five main elements (Fig. 12.1).

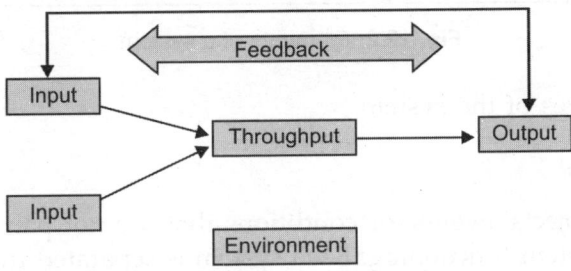

Fig. 12.1: Elements of systems theory

Elements

1. Input
2. Output
3. Throughput
4. Feedback
5. Environment

Classic System Elements

The elements of any system are: (Fig. 12.2)
- Goal
- Environment
- Input
- Process or throughput
- Output

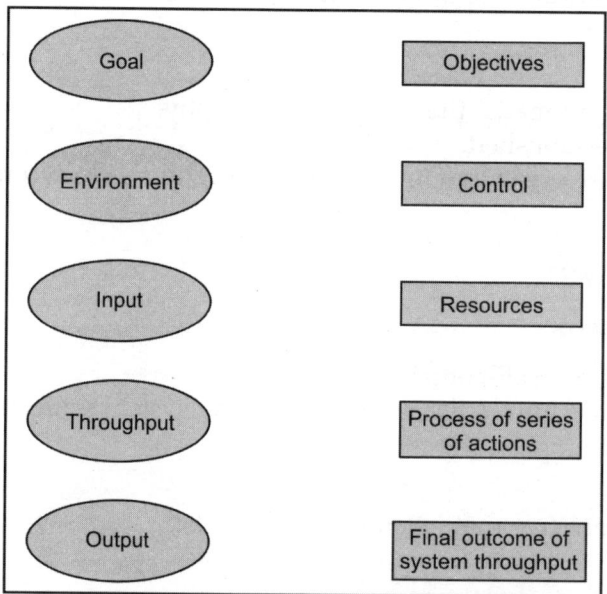

Fig. 12.2: Elements of a system

Goal: Is the objectives of the system.

Environment/Control

Defined as set of objects, events, or conditions that are not part of the system, but has a bearing on system functioning. Each system is separated from its environment by the system boundary.

Input is the energizer and operating materials of the system. This consists of information, money, energy, time, effort or raw materials.

Input for nursing system are people like nurses, clerks, auxiliaries, equipment such as thermometer, BP apparatus, syringes, etc. supplies such as dressings, linen, lotions used in providing care and comfort to patients, in addition, nursing theory, research findings, nursing interventions.

Throughput: It is the process of series of actions by which system converts input from the environment into product and services that are usable by the system itself or by the environment.

In nursing the patient care process where patients are to move from impaired, dependent state to a more whole and independent state and protects others from unnecessary loss of comfort, strength and integrity as they get informed. Also the state development process where employees are brought from lower to higher levels of knowledge and skill through coaching and education further the research program where employees discover methods for improving patients care and health promotion.

Output is the final outcome of systems throughput. The product or service nursing department outputs are improved vital signs, improved activities of daily living, increased comfort, improved self-care knowledge and increased satisfaction of care. Other outputs include the research reports, increased knowledge and skills.

Feedback and Control

Feedback is information about some aspects of data or energy processing that can be used to monitor and evaluate system performance and guide it to move effective performance.

Controls

They are actions taken by system operations to regulate input, process or output elements so as to improve system functions.

For example
- Control over *throughput regulates* the time, efficiency and safety operations.
- Control over *output regulates* production quality and quantity.

Systems Analysis

It is a scientific and detailed definition of a system that, it examines:
- The systems purpose.
- Overall requirements.
- Number and types of subsystem.
- Nature of subsystem interactions.

Basic Principles of System Approach to Nursing Management

There are 13 principles.
1. It requires investigating the whole situation.
2. Each system behaves in a characteristic manner because of the unique relationships among its path.
3. Each system is self contained entity but also part of an other system.
4. System maintenance is the central objective of most organizations.
5. Every system is an information system.
6. Although boundary divides the system from its environment, system theory says that an open system from its environments is highly inter-related.
7. System approach requires a situation be viewed as a whole, but highly complex system may be broken into subsystems so that each can be analyzed and understood.
8. System consists of objects and their relationships. Relationships are more important for the functioning of the system.
9. A system is dynamic network of connecting elements. A change in one element produces change in all the elements.
10. When subsystems are arranged in series, as when output of one system becomes input for another, process alterations in any system necessitate alterations in other related subsystems.
11. Changes in system boundary usually alter the function of selected subsystems and total system output.
12. All systems lend toward equilibrium, a balance of various forces operating within and on the system.
13. To function smoothly a system must be goal directed, governed by feedback and capable of adapting to changes in the external circumstances.

Advantages and Disadvantages of Systems Approach (Table 12.1)

What is the significance of systems theory to the nurse manager?

Nurse manager works ....within a system.
- Nursing department is a ....**functional system.**
- The nursing process is a............information and **service system.**
- Management process is a........**power system.**
- Nursing procedures and protocols......mental motor work system.
- Each employee that they supervise is........ **personality system.**
- The group that they lead is ....**social system.**

Table 12.1: Advantages and Disadvantages of system

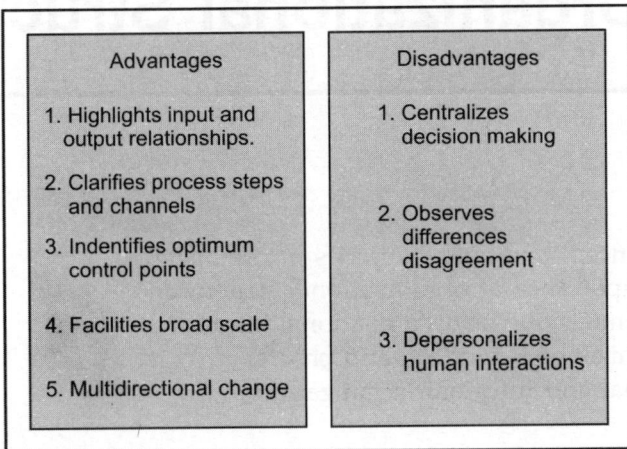

Why Nurse Managers Need to know the Systems Approach?

- It is helpful in evaluating the nursing departments effectiveness.
- It enables managers to contrasts cost of system inputs and value system of outputs.

The nurse manager must know the systems approach as this terminology is used by other disciplines and to integrate the principles in the management.

13 Organizational Structure

OBJECTIVES

1. Explain the concept and characteristics of organization.
2. Discuss the importance of organizational structure.
3. Identify the dimensions of organizational structure.
4. Describe organizational models, and charts.
5. Compare formal and informal organization.

INTRODUCTION

The term organization is used in the management in **two different ways.**
1. Organization as a structure.
2. Organization as a process.

Organization Structure, as *a structure*

- Organization is the network of **Horizontal and vertical** relationships among the members of a group designed to accomplish some of common objectives.
- It is a system of **formal relationships** that govern the activities of people.
- The horizontal dimension depicts differentiation **of jobs into department's or divisions.**
- The vertical dimension reflects the hierarchy of **authority relationships** with a numbers of levels from top to bottom.

Organization as Process

Organizing is continuous and dynamic process of creating harmonious authority-responsibility relationships between specialized units.

The end result of organization process is *Organizational structure.*

Importance of Organization Structure

1. It is the foundation upon which the whole structure of management is built.
2. It is the backbone of the management.
3. Sound organization can contribute greatly to the success of an institution.

Which are the ways an organization can contribute to success of an institution?
- Facilitates administration.
- Facilitates growth and diversification.
- Permits optimum use of technological improvements.
- Encourages use of human beings.
- Stimulates creativity.

The dimensions of an organizational structure

Dimensions
1. Standardization: For example, Department policy
2. Centralization of authority: For example, Chain of accountability
3. Specialization: For example, Financial duties
4. Communication: For example, Transmission of information
5. Innovation: For example, Commitment to implement research findings.

ORGANIZATIONAL MODELS

The most common models include (Fig. 13.1):

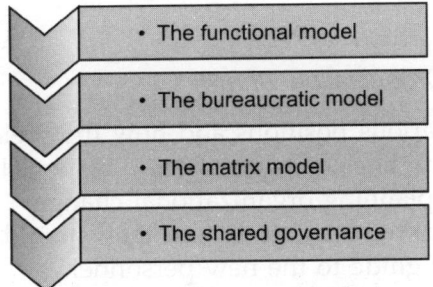

Fig. 13.1: Organizational Models

Types of Organizations

- Formal organization
- Informal organization

Formal Organization

It refers to:
- A pattern of activities
- Process human relationships
- Roles planned and structured in order to accomplish organizational goals.

Informal Organization

It refers to:
- The pattern of activities
- Interactions
- Human relationships.

Which emerge spontaneously due to social and psychological forces operating at work place.

ORGANIZATION CHARTS

An organization chart is a graphic portrayal of the various positions in the organization and the formal relationships among them. It server as a blue print.

Types of Organization Charts

There are many. But all the organization charts are classified into *two broad categories*.
1. *Vertical charts:*
   - This is called top to down chart.
   - Lowest position is shown at the bottom. It is most widely used.
2. *Horizontal charts*
   - This is called left to right chart.
   - Highest position is placed at extreme right and the lowest is at the extreme left.

Advantages or Uses of Organization Chart

- It shows clearly the various positions and how they relate to one another.
- It shows at a glance the lines of authority and responsibility.
- It provides a basis of planning organizational change.
- It provides guidance to outsiders to whom they should contact.
- It serves as a valuable guide to the new personnel.
- It helps to point out inconsistencies and deficiencies.
- It provides a framework for classification and evaluation of personnel.
- It provides clues to the lines of promotion.
- It also facilitates communication.

Principles of Organization Charts

- Should have a *clear title*.
- Should clearly show the *lines of authority*.
- Positions of *equal ranks* must be shown at the *same level*.
- *Solid lines* must be used to indicate the line of authority.
- Staff relationships by *dotted lines*.
- Complete chart should be on a *single sheet*.
- *Colors* may be used to indicate *different departments*.

Limitations

- Fails to recognize informal relationships.
- Does not represent flexibility.
- It introduces bureaucratic rigidity in the formal relationships.
- Shows the relationships which is supposed to exist rather than what actually exist.
- Fail to show how much authority and responsibility an individual can exercise due to over simplification.
- Poorly designed charts cause confusion and misunderstanding.
- They may create superiority and inferiority feelings and lead to conflicts in the organization.

Line-staff Organization

This is a pattern in which the line-staff at higher level is provided with advisory or consultative staff.
- Though they are consultative staff, they are at higher level.
- Directly under the control of line managers.
- Shown at the side of line manager marked with dotted lines or solid lines.

Unit VI: Patient Care Management

14 Management of Hospital Departments

OBJECTIVES

1. Describe the concept and functions of the hospital.
2. Discuss the hospital classifications and organization.
3. Describe the major departments.

INTRODUCTION

In the past, the hospital has been a place for care of the sick. Today, the hospital has become a center of technical services for the sick and well, inpatients as well as outpatients with greater emphasis on achieving the highest standards of patient care and community health.

DEFINITION

A hospital is an institution with the primary function of providing diagnostic and therapeutic patient services for a variety of medical conditions, both medical and surgical.

A hospital is a health care institution with an organized medical and professional staff, and with permanent facilities that include inpatient beds, provides medical, nursing and other health related services to patients.

FUNCTIONS OF THE HOSPITAL

1. *Patient care:* Primary function (curative function) refers to any type of care given to patients by the health team members, e.g. physicians, nurses, physical therapist, dietitians, etc. It also includes health teaching to patients.
2. *Health personnel education:* Secondary function (educational function) refers to the education of professional and technical personnel who provide health services, e.g. physicians, nurses, dentists, therapist, technicians, etc.
3. *Health promotion:* Secondary function (preventive function) an emerging function for the hospital is that of a community health center taking an active role to improve the health of the population it serves. Hospitals as major community health centers can sponsor programs of environmental and occupational health, home care services, etc.
4. *Health related research:* Secondary function (Research-function) Research that focuses on the improvement of health and/or prevention of disease.

CLASSIFICATION OF HOSPITALS

Hospitals are classified according to:

The Type of Service

There are two groups of hospitals: General and Special.

009General Hospitals

They care for patients with various disease conditions for both sexes to all ages, medical, surgical, pediatrics, obstetrics, eye and ear hospital, etc.

General hospitals may contain specialized units staffed by specialized personnel, Renal unit, Intensive Care Unit, Coronary Care Unit, Plastic Surgery Unit and Burn Unit. There may be specialization at unit level, Neurological, Urological, Orthopedic units, etc.

Special Hospitals

They limit their service to a particular condition, orthopedic, maternity, pediatrics, geriatrics, etc.

Administration, Ownership, Control or Financial Income

Governmental or Public Hospital

They are owned, administered and controlled by the Government. They provide free care for patients. They may offer private accommodation for fee-paying patients. The Governmental hospitals are owned by:
- The Ministry of Health or State Government
- The University or Central Government, e.g. Railways, Defense
- Others: Quasi Government.

Non-Governmental or Private

They depend on:
- **Proprietary:** Privately owned or controlled by an individual or group of physicians or citizens or by private organization (profit-making).
- **Voluntary:** Owned and operated by nonprofit organization, i.e. mosque or church authorities.

Length of Stay

Hospitals are classified depending on the duration of stay.

Short-term or Short-stay Hospitals

These are hospitals where over 90% of all patients admitted stay less than 30 days, e.g. sub-divisional or small hospitals.

Long-term or Long-stay Hospitals

These are hospitals where over 90% of all patients admitted and stay 30 days or more, e.g. mental health centers.

Type of Medical Staff

Some hospitals are classified according to the type of medical personnel available.

Closed-staff Hospital

Physicians are held responsible for all medical activities in the hospital including the diagnosis and treatment of patient-fee paying and emergency.

Open-staff Hospital

This type of hospital permits other physicians in the community to admit and treat patients.

Size or Bed Capacity

Depending on the capacity of the beds the hospitals may be classified as:
- Small hospitals are with the capacity of 100 beds or less.
- Medium size hospital is with the capacity with 100 to 300 beds.
- Large hospitals are with the capacity 300 to 1000 beds.

The Area Served

For example: Primary health centers, subcenters, etc.

ORGANIZATION OF THE HOSPITAL

At the head of any hospital organization there is a governing board or board of directors (policy-making body) which represents the owners.

Authority for the administration of the hospital is delegated by the governing board to the director or administrator. The administrator is responsible for maintaining standards of service and patient care established by the board. He is responsible to carry out the functions of the hospital in accordance with the philosophy and established policies set by the governing board. He delegates the responsibility for the different departments to the department heads who are specialist in their field. In large hospitals, the administrator has one or more assistants to help with the administration of various departments (Fig. 14.1).

Hospital Health Service Departments (Table 14.1)

The hospital areas are divided into two major departments. They are professional health service departments and non-professional health service departments.

Management of Hospital Departments

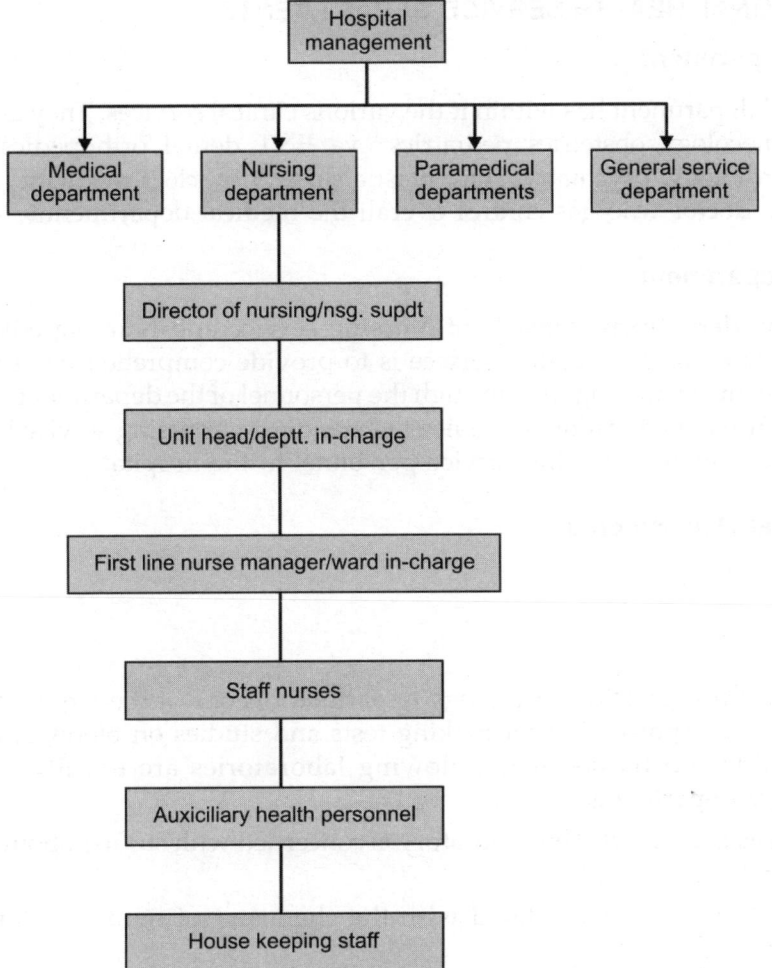

Fig. 14.1: Nursing administration structure

Table 14.1: Hospital health service departments

Professional health service departments	Non-professional health service departments
Medical department	Admitting department
Nursing department	Personnel department
Paramedical departments	Purchase department
• Laboratory	Medical records
Pharmacy department	Accounts (business office)
Physical medicine and rehabilitation department	House-keeping department
Radiology department	Laundry department
Dietary department (catering)	Mechanical department
Out-patient department	Maintenance department
• Accident and emergency department (A and E)	Central sterile supply department (CSSD)
	Social service department/public relation department

PROFESSIONAL HEALTH SERVICE DEPARTMENTS

Medical Department

The medical department has within it the various clinical services. They are: medicine, surgery, gynecology, obstetrics, pediatrics, eye, ENT, dental, orthopedics, neurology, urology, cardiology, psychiatry, skin, plastic surgery, nuclear medicine, etc. medical director is a doctor who gas control overall the medical department.

Nursing Department

The Nursing department consists of Nursing service and Nursing education. The primary purpose of the Nursing service is to provide comprehensive, safe, effective and well-organized nursing care through the personnel of the department. The primary purpose of nursing education is to raise the standard of nursing service by providing in service education to nursing service personnel in the hospital.

Paramedical Departments

They include:

Laboratory

a. *Pathology department:* The pathology department is one of the largest departments and has the responsibility for making tests and studies on blood, sputum, feces, body fluids and tissues. The following laboratories are usually found in the pathology department.
b. *Bacteriology department:* This laboratory is concerned with studies about the bacteria and their toxins.
c. *Biochemistry:* This is considered with the chemistry of living organisms and of vital processes.
d. *Hematology laboratory:* It is responsible for making hemoglobin determinations, coagulation time studies, red and white cell counts and special blood pathology studies for anemia and leukemia, etc.
e. *Parasitological laboratory:* It studies the presence of parasites, the cyst and ova of the parasites that are found in the feces.
f. *Serology laboratory:* It does blood agglutination tests, Wassermann tests, VD.
g. *Blood bank:* It has the responsibility for collecting and processing all blood used in the hospital for transfusions. It makes studies on newborn infants who may have hemolytic diseases, and does antibody studies on the prenatal patients.
h. *Histopathology laboratory:* It prepares tissues for gross and microscopic studies.

Small hospitals which do not have a pathology department send specimens to be investigated to a central pathology service or to a large hospital.

Pharmacy Department

The pharmacy department has the responsibility for selecting, purchasing, compounding, storing and dispensing all drugs and medications for in-patients and outpatients. The pharmacy should be under the supervision of registered pharmacist.

Physical Medicine and Rehabilitation Department

This department treats patients who have functional disabilities resulting from disease condition or injuries. It has several specialties such as: physical therapy, occupational therapy, speech therapy and vocational training. This department is under the direction of a well-qualified physician who has special training in the field of physical medicine and rehabilitation. The staff should include therapist with qualification in the various specialties. The work of this department is one part of the total patient care plan.

Radiology Department

This department functions under the control of radiologist and qualified technical staff. It has the following diagnostic and therapeutic services for inpatients and outpatients.
- Radiographic examination and their interactions.
- X-ray, radium, radioactive cobalt and other radioactive therapy.
- Radioactive isotopes tracer.
- Radioactive isotopes therapy.

Dietary Department (Catering)

In most hospitals, this department is under the direction of a trained dietitian. The department is charged with:
a. Ordering and preparation of food.
b. Tray service.
c. Diet teaching.

The dietitian is a member of the health team and works closely with nursing service personnel in meeting the patient's nutritional needs and in teaching. He/she is responsible for the ordering of supplies and the supervision of all staff engaged in the preparation and delivery of food.

The kitchen should have ample light and air and should be as close as possible to the stairs, the dining rooms and the elevators.

Procedures for handling dishes for communicable disease patients should be separated from general patients.

Milk purchase and service should adhere to sanitary regulations, procured from an approved source, pasteurized and served to patients in individual sealed containers.

A periodic complete physical examination including X-ray of chest, analysis of stool and urine and should be consider in order to detect silent carriers and take appropriate action. Daily inspection of personal appearance and hygiene also are important.

Three types of dietary service are in use:
a. Centralized service.
b. Decentralized service.
c. A combination of (a) and (b).

Outpatient Department

This is a combination of several departments. It is a miniature of the hospital except that the patients are ambulatory. Services are provided by specialists. Individuals may attend this department for the purpose of receiving treatment, or to enable a physician to assess their progress following discharge from hospital.

Accident and Emergency Department (A + E)

In most large hospitals, people who are classified as "emergency admissions" are received into this department to receive lifesaving services immediately needed after thorough examination by the responsible physician, i.e. road accidents, people who become suddenly very ill, etc. Arrangements for admission to hospital are made if necessary.

Some accident and emergency departments have their own operating room where minor surgery can be performed, a plaster room where plaster casts are applied, and other services, such as X-ray and pharmacy.

Operating Theater

Depending on the size of the hospital, there may be one or more number of operating rooms. In addition to the rooms where surgery is performed, there are: sterilizing rooms, anesthetic rooms, recovery rooms, utility and storage rooms, staff amenities such as offices, toilets, etc.

In addition to these departments mentioned, large hospitals may provide other services such as intensive care, education department, blood bank, referral services to other hospital, etc.

NON-PROFESSIONAL HEALTH SERVICE DEPARTMENTS (BUSINESS MANAGEMENT)

Admitting Department

This department has the responsibility for admitting the patient to the hospital. It should maintain good public relations. The patient, family and friends must be treated with utmost respect, courtesy and tact. Appropriate answers are to be given upon enquiries about the hospital.

Personnel Department (Functions)

a. Recruitment of personnel.
b. Interviewing.
c. Promotion and transfer.

d. Termination of employment.
e. In-service training.
f. Safety.
g. Health programs.
h. Recreation.
i. Remuneration and incentives.

Purchase Department

This department has the responsibility for purchasing all supplies and equipment for the hospital.

Medical Records

This is one of the important departments in the hospital. The patients records (charts, X-ray, etc.) are valuable not only to the patient but also to the doctor and to medical and nursing education and research.

Accounts (Business Office)

This department has the responsibility for collecting the money which is owed to the hospital, paying for supplies and equipment, handling all records pertaining to hospital finance, assisting with budget, etc.

Housekeeping Department (Domestic Services)

This department's main function is to keep the hospital clean. It plays an important role in hospital hygiene and infection control.

Laundry Department

The laundry takes care of the entire linen of the hospital. It has the responsibility of washing, repairing and replacing linen. The location should be as far as possible from patient services areas to reduce noise. Linen which requires special care should be marked before it is sent to the laundry. Nursing personnel should be careful and alert the laundry workers to the centralization of laundry service promote efficient and quick service.

Mechanical Department

Electricity, water supply, heat, air conditioning, etc. are looked after by the mechanical department.

Maintenance Department

The maintenance department keeps the hospital in good condition. Carpenters, painters, gardeners, etc. are included in the personnel of this department.

Central Sterile Supply Department (CSSD)

In modern hospitals, the trend is toward centralization of preparation and sterilization of supplies and equipment. The location should be as central as possible within the hospital with ample light. Where space conditions permit, this department should adjoin the operating department since it uses a large amount of surgical supplies.

Purpose

i. To prepare and furnish other departments and nursing units with sterile equipment and supplies needed in the patient care.
ii. To ensure:
   a. Standardization, and better utilization and control of supplies and equipment used foe diagnosis and treatment.
   b. More adequate methods of sterilization than on a nursing unit.
   c. Early detection of mechanical defects in equipment through regular checks.
   d. Economy of time and better care.

Modern hospitals use elevator between the CSSD and nursing units. Items not used within 7 to 10 days should be resterilized.

Social Service Department/Public Relation Department

This department assists in obtaining financial aid for patients and their families. It advises on the agencies through which help of various kinds can be arranged. It serves as a liaison between the patient and community agencies.

Class Exercise

Analyze organizational structure in the unit/department.

Purpose

To help the students.
- Identify the organizational structure of the hospital and decide whether the principles of organization are implemented in the structure identified and to analyze the best suited organizational type for nursing among the basic organizational types used in health care system.
- To exercise critical thinking to conceptualize and analyze possible solutions to a practical experience incident.

Directions

Divide the students into groups of (6-8) as theory starts; to collect the relevant information. Each group works individually.

Exercise to Students

Obtain an organizational chart from your clinical unit. Discuss whether the principles of organization are implemented in the structure.

15
Management of Nursing Services

NURSING CARE DELIVERY SYSTEM

Objectives

1. Describe the organizational structure and classification of nursing service personnel.
2. Discuss the functions of nursing practice department.
3. Describe the concept and functions of the nursing unit.
4. Discuss the types of nursing units and unit organization.
5. Describe the nursing unit environment.

The Nursing Practice Department

The nursing department is the largest department in the hospital. The head of department is the director of nursing (the nursing administrator, matron, nursing officer). She is responsible directly to the hospital administrator for the efficient management of the department. She / he have at least on assistant for each period of the day since the nursing department serves 24 hours.

The director of nursing delegates the management of two or more nursing units within the hospital to a nurse supervisor who in turn delegates the management of the nursing unit to the first line nurse manager (Head nurse "HN") (Fig. 15.1). The first-line nurse manager (Head nurse "HN"), in turn delegates the care of the patients to the unit staff.

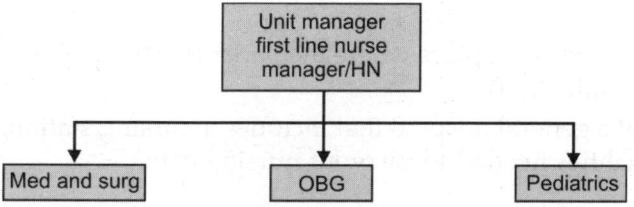

Fig. 15.1: Unit–organization structure

Classification of Nursing Practice Personnel

The department consists of two main classifications:
  a. **Professional nursing personnel:**
   They are director, assistants, supervisors, first-line managers (HN) and staff nurses.

b. Non-professional nursing personnel:
They are practical nurses (assistant nurses), nurses aides, orderlies and clerks.

Function of the Nursing Department

- To plan, provide and evaluate nursing care for patient and families.
- To define and implement the philosophy, objectives and standards for nursing care of the patients.
- To provide and implement a departmental plan of administrative authority which delineates responsibilities and duties of each category of nursing personnel.
- To coordinate the functions of the department with the functions of all other departments.
- To estimate the requirements of the department.
- To interpret hospital and nursing practice objectives to the patients and community.
- To participate in the formulation of personnel policies, to implement established policies and evaluate their effectiveness.
- To develop an effective system of nursing records and reports.
- To estimate needs for facilities, supplies and equipment.
- To participate in financial planning.
- To participate in studies and research projects for the improvement of patient care and hospital services.
- To provide and implement continuing education program for all nursing personnel.
- To participate in and or facilitate all educational programs of students in the health care field.

The Nursing Unit / Ward

The nursing unit is referred to as the inpatient care unit, or the hospital unit or ward.

Definition

The nursing unit/ward is the place where the patients actually live during their stay in the hospital (hospitalization).

It is a section of a general hospital that includes a nursing station, the beds it serves and associated facilities needed to carryout nursing care.

Specific Functions of Nursing Unit

- Provide and maintain the highest quality patient care with the lowest possible cost.
- Furnish the most desirable environment (safe, comfortable and pleasant) for patients and health service personnel, i.e. medical and nursing staff as well as the other hospital personnel.
- Consider needs of patients families and significant others.

- Provide adequate space to facilitate the carrying out of all the activities needed, i.e. using different types of equipment with minimum waste of personnel time, i.e. wide doors and corridors, wheel chair with IV stand, patient movement in their beds with attached apparatus → improves quality care.
- Promote job satisfaction of the health personnel.

TYPE OF NURSING UNITS

General Units

Where there are similar medical or surgical treatments, e.g. medical or surgical units.

Special units: they are designed according to:

a. Patients age, e.g. pediatrics, geriatrics, etc.
b. Patients needs, e.g. recovery room, nursery, intensive care unit, etc.
c. Medical specialty, e.g. neurosurgery, gynecology, dermatology, ophthalmology, etc. patient behavior, e.g. psychiatry.

Recently, a system known as progressive patient care (5 PPC) has been adopted in some hospitals-intensive care unit (ICU), intermediate-care unit, self-care unit, long-term care unit and home-care unit. This system is one of organizing the hospital units around the medical needs of patients and grouping them according to their degree of illness and their needs of nursing care.

Though it is advantageous in terms of economy of manpower and material, it has failed to sustain practically due to the current trends in specialization and super specialization.

Unit Organization

Central hospitals in omen, the first-line manager (ward nurse/senior nurse) directs the operation of the nursing unit. The first-line nurse manager delegates the care of patients to the unit staff utilizing to the fullest, the skills of each. She/he gives them direct supervision guidance and teaching. She/he is responsible to the principal nursing officer/matron through Nursing Officer (NO) of the unit and her/his deputy. She/he is indirectly responsible to the Head of the Nursing Affairs (HNA) and the Director of Nursing Affairs (DNA).

In Regional Hospitals the first-line nurse manager (the senior nurse) is the in-charge of the Nursing unit. She/he is responsible to the Nursing Officer (Matron) through the nurse supervisor for the efficient management of the nursing unit. Mean while she/he is responsible indirectly to the Head of Nursing Affairs (HNA) of the region. The nursing unit staff are directly responsible to the first-line nurse manager (Senior Nurse). They include staff nurses, Assistant/Practical nurses, Nurse's aids and medical orderlies. They are responsible to the supervisor and to the Nursing Officer (Matron) through the first-line nurse manager.

Nursing Unit Environment

1. The nursing unit environment is made up of two basic components.
2. The physical component; furniture, furnishing, lighting, etc.

The psychosocial component; created by the customs, cultural values, norms and interpersonal relationships existing in the nursing unit. It influences the patient's reaction to illness, and can play a role in his / her recovery and well-being. Therefore, the provision of a safe, comfortable and pleasant unit environment should be the aim of unit personnel and every member of the health team.

ESSENTIAL AREAS AND FACILITIES IN THE NURSING UNIT

The Nurse's Station

It is placed at the entrance of the nursing unit or as centrally as possible to command a wide view of the unit. It is used for office work, handling patients calls. Keeping charts, etc.

Near the nurses station there should be a conference room, a treatment room, medicine closet, toilet room and handwashing facilities for staff.

Closets

Medicine closet for 24 hr distribution of medicines to patients, storage closet for the storage of equipment and supplies used in nursing procedures, linen closet for the storage of clean linen, janitors closet or cleaners room to store the equipment needed for unit cleaning.

Rooms

The patient's room, examining room and treatment room, utility room, visitors room, conference and classrooms, doctors room consulting offices, nurse in-charge office, unit laboratory, serving kitchen, toilet-bath unit, laundry and waste chutes.

The Patient Rooms

There are three types in each hospital unit:
1. Private or single rooms (one bed room), most expensive. The patient will have his own room, bath and toilet to secure comfort and privacy.
2. Semi-private: two bedrooms or double or less expensive.
3. General wards: More than two, 6-8 or 10 beds in each room. Least expensive either for patients who are charged less or free.

Physical factors:
- Adequate lighting during day and night.
- Adequate ventilation without causing draughts and free from un pleasant odors.
- Comfortable temperature and free from noise.
- Cleanliness of all surface and furnishing that the individual is likely to handle.
- Immediate removal of equipment used, for cleaning purposes.
- Provision for the disposal of refuse and excreta.

PATIENT CLASSIFICATION SYSTEM

Objectives

1. Explain the importance of patient classification system for nursing management.
2. Identify the key characteristics of a patient classification system.
3. Differentiate between the types of patient classification system.
4. Enumerate the care descriptors commonly used in patient classification.
5. Describe diagnostic related groups (DRG).

Introduction

Patient classification, staffing, and scheduling and strategies used in the delivery of patient care. These reflect sensitive to cost containment, length of hospitalization and improvement of patient care.

Importance of Patient Classification

Patient classification system (PCS) provides a method of quantitatively estimating and assessing patient needs in relation to nursing care. It is a way of determining the amount and type of care of a patient requires as well as providing a means of standardizing nursing care practice.

As economic issues have become important health care decision making, patient classification system (PSC) provides an input in how nursing care is delivered, the amount of time required, the cost involved and evaluates the cost-efficient and cost effective care. PCS can be used as a valid and reliable instrument to measure the acuity level of patients in terms of nursing workload and number of nursing staff needed as well as variation in nursing care. This helps to simplify staff allocation and scheduling. This system can also be used effectively for long range staffing, budgeting, management planning, quality management programs, compliance with licensing and industry standards and regulations.

Purpose of Patient Classification System

It is a scheme for grouping patients according to the amount and complexity of their nursing care requirements. The purpose of PCS is to assess patients, group them with patients having similar needs and assign patients in each group, a numerical score to quantify their nursing care needs.

Types of Patient Classification System

1. *Factor evaluation system:* Patient needs are scored on multiple care descriptors.
2. *Prototype evaluation system:* Describes typical patient and varying need levels.
3. *Diagnostic related groups (DRG):* Grouping patients for prospective payment.

Factor Evaluation System

Most of the health care agencies use this PCS where several care elements or descriptors are identified, each element is divided into subelements and a standard time is determined for accomplishing each subelement.

The descriptors used to measure patients dependency needs are activities of daily living: feeding, grooming, toileting, comport measures and mobility. The required to assist a patient with each activity is quantified from the least amount of time required to the greatest amount of time required. For example, as feeds self–as requires tube feeding.

Common Care Descriptors

Hygiene, nutrition, medications, fluid management, skin and wound care, respiratory care, circulatory care, elimination, mobility, special diagnostic and treatment procedures, health teaching and daily activities of living.

After care descriptors have been selected, the levels of care, intensity is defined for each descriptor. The level is differentiated by the amount of nursing time and frequency of each care measure.

1. The factor system is referred to as objective because specifying particular indicators or factors associated with patient care helps to ensure objectivity by the rater.
2. Prototype evaluation system: This is considered subjective and uses broad descriptive categories to describe the patient and needs. Characteristics are listed for a typical patient in each of the categories.

Category I

Patients with acute, episodic disease or disability who will return to their pre-illness level to functioning and for whom the goal is to relieve existing health problem.

Category II

Patients with chronic disease with acute episode of illness but has potential to return to pre-episodic level of functioning where the chronic health problem can be managed by self or the family.

Category III

Patients with chronic disease where return to pre-illness level of functioning but potential to increase level of functioning with care goal is rehabilitation to a maximum level of functioning with agency support.

Category IV

Patients with chronic disease who cannot be maintained at home without ongoing agency support.

Category V

Patient with end stage of illness. However, the most effective patient classification system is one that is specifically tailored to the clinical situation where it will be used.

Diagnostic Related Groups (DGR)

This is prospective payment system. It has set a predetermined price for patient hospital care of medicare recipients according to the patient's placement in one of 467 diagnostic related groups. The DRG system is a strategy for grouping patients according to demographic, diagnostic and therapeutic characteristics that correlate with their use of hospital facilities.

Under this prospective payment system hospitals are paid a fixed price for all inpatients, according to the DRG into which he/she is classified at time of discharge from the hospital. If the hospital cost for the patient care is less than the fixed rate, the hospital gets profit. If the cost exceeds the fixed rate, the hospital is at loss. DGR system provides incentive for early hospital discharge but the quality of care is affected.

Patient classification system looks at various kinds of nursing activities to determine patient care requirements. So it is essential that as many categories as possible be considered. A patient classification system assists in identifying individual patient care requirements and can be instrumental in facilitating the equitable distribution of time and personnel.

THE ROLE OF NURSE MANAGER

Objectives

1. Identify the roles of the nurse manager.
2. Discuss the management levels.
3. Describe the concept and role of the first line manager in the nursing unit.

Introduction

Professional and non-professional nursing service personnel have different roles to play in the nursing unit. *A role is appropriate behavior which goes with a position*. The atmosphere of the nursing unit created by the behavior of the first line nurse manager or head nurse and will affect the attitude of unit nursing personnel and in turn their roles in giving quality patient care.

ROLES AND RESPONSIBILITIES

There are *six main roles* and functions of the nurse manager listed by *American organization of nurse executives (AONE)*

1. The nurse manager is accountable for excellence in the clinical practice of nursing and the delivery of patient care on a selected unit or area within the health care institutions.
2. The nurse manager is accountable for managing human, fiscal and other resources needed to a manage clinical nursing practice and patient care.
3. The nurse manager is accountable for facilitating development of licensed and unlicensed nursing and health care personnel.
4. The nurse manager is accountable for ensuring institutional compliance with professional, regulatory, and government standards of care.

5. The nurse manager is accountable for planning as it relates to the units or areas, department, and organization as a whole.
6. The nurse manager is accountable for facilitating cooperative and collaborative relationship among disciplines / departments to ensure effective delivery of quality care.

Levels of Management (Fig. 15.2)

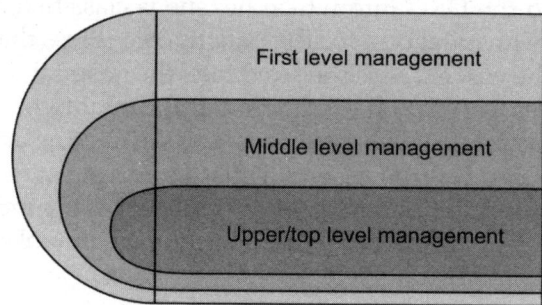

Fig. 15.2: Three levels of management

First Level Management

The first line manager is responsible for supervising the work of non-managerial personnel and the day-to-day activities of a specific work unit or units.
The manager is responsible for:
- Clinical nursing practice,
- Patient care delivery,
- Use of human,
- Fiscal and other resources,
- Personnel development,
- Compliance with regulatory and professional standards,
- Fostering interdisciplinary collaborative relationships, and
- Strategic planning.

Middle Level Management

Middle level managers are supervisory level staff engaged in supervising the first-line nurse managers of particular specialty. For example, medical unit may have number of wards, such as male and female medical wards, pediatric medical wards MICU, etc. or in a given geographic area. For example, Surgical floor / first floor, second floor, etc. of a hospital.

Upper/Top Level Management

The Nurse Director is responsible for managing the Nursing Department in the hospital. All middle level managers report to her/him regarding the matters related to their specified units.

FIRST-LINE NURSE MANAGER (HEAD NURSE)

Definition

The first-line nurse manager (Head nurse) is a nurse who is responsible for the management of the activities in a single nursing unit.

First-line nurse manager assumes three main functional areas of responsibilities namely:
1. Patient care management,
2. Staff management, and
3. Nursing unit management.

Patient Care Management

The application of nursing process:
a. **Assess and analyze patient's needs and develop the plan of care to meet needs.**
   - Determine nursing diagnosis.
   - Determine the priorities to the diagnosed problems.
   - Select objectives for nursing.
   - Record nursing orders and develop the patient care plan.
   - Set standards to evaluate the quality and quantity of patient care.

   For example, procedure manual, unit policies, job descriptions, and standard nursing care.

b. **Assignment of personnel to meet patient needs:**
   Assignment refers to written delegation of duties in the care of patient by trained personnel employed in the unit.

Purpose

- To delegate the work to be done to unit nursing staff.
- To gain the cooperation of the unit nursing staff by knowing and accepting the work to be done.

Principles of Assignment

1. Assignment should be made for each individual nurse.
2. Assignment should be based on:
   - The abilities, interests, previous experience, knowledge, skills of each individual nurse to ensure maximum utilization of their unique talents and abilities.
   - The personal qualities of the individual nurses as some nurses may relate better than others to some patients, for example, more patience adolescent with young nurse, etc.
   - Patients needs and problems.
   - Job description a detailed account of roles and responsibilities in a given designation / position, given to all the employees on employment.
3. Assignment should be balanced among nursing staff and should consider;
   - The amount of time necessary to give nursing care indicated.

- What activity is more urgent (priority setting).
- The meeting of predictable (lab-investigations, X-ray) and non-predictable events (emergencies as they arise, e.g. sudden changes in patient condition).
- Availability of supplies, equipment (centralized or decentralized).
4. Assign the individual nurse to the same patient as long as practical to ensure continuity of patient care.
5. Provide necessary information and explanations concerning the assignment of duties before they carry them out.
6. Put assignment in writing, simple, clear, and easily understood to serve as a guide.
7. Check to see that the entire work–load is covered with no overlapping of assignments. Two workers should never be assigned to the same task.

Types of Assignments

- Patient care assignment
- Unit care assignments

Patient Care Assignments: Patient care assignments further classified in to;
- Individual assignments
- Team assignments.

Individual assignments: Individual patient care is the ideal which promotes the quality patient care and accountability of nurses for the welfare of the patient, better follow up on the prognosis and decision making abilities.

Advantages: It is advantages to the patients to have better communication and approach to the care provider, gains confidence to share his health and psychosocial problems to the nurse, hence make the hospital stay comfortable.

Team assignment: The activities of routine patient care are carried out by the nurses in order to complete the routines.
Example: Vital signs may be checked for all the patients by one nurse, medication by an other, attending rounds by an other nurse, etc. the work may be assigned by the in-charge according to the seniority or experience of the nurses on the shift.

Advantages
- The patient care can be completed on time during the shift.
- Can be managed when there is shortage of nurses.
- When staff nurses from other unit are pulled in to help in emergencies.

Unit care Assignments: The in-charge nurse can give special assignments related to the unit management depending on the seniority and efficiency of nurses working along with her, delegating some of her responsibilities like inventory of narcotics, emergency trolley equipment, linen, daily utility equipment, treatment room, setting up of admission records, etc.

c. **Supervise all Nursing activities related to direct and indirect patient care:**
Conduct's rounds during the day by self, with unit staff and with physician.

1. **Rounds by self:**
Purposes

- To observe all the patients and talk to them.
- Observe general condition, physical appearance, facial expression, color, skin condition, pulse, respiration, complaints, condition of wounds, accuracy of documentation, progress, satisfaction of care provided, etc.
- To assess the adequacy of nursing care given based on the standards set by each member of the nursing staff, offer necessary guidance and teaching.
- To check different records for adequacy, completeness and legibility, etc.
- To assess the environment for cleanliness, orderliness, light, ventilation, control of noise, defective/shortage of equipment, emergency equipment, safety, privacy, etc.

2. **Rounds with unit nursing staff:**
Purposes

- To observe health education given to the patients, assess their progress and to discuss needed intervention.
- To promote good interpersonal relationship with unit staff by showing interest in them.
- To assess the adequacy of nursing care given by the nursing staff and give necessary assistance if needed.
- To receive information about the patients education from the assigned nurse and any difficulties encountered.

3. **Rounds with the physician:**
Purposes

- To exchange information concerning patients condition and progress in the presence of an assigned nurse.
- To receive new orders.
- Hold short conference with the nursing staff before the days work begins to be sure that each staff member understand she/his assignment.

d. **Participate in patient education and rehabilitation.**
- Allays fears of hospitalization.
- Inform the patient about hospital policies and regulations.
- Explain available services.
- Be sure that explanations are given for each procedure before performing and teaching plans are formulated and implemented based on patients needs.

Staff Management

There are different categories of unit nursing staff with variation in education and experience. The nurse in charge is responsible for their development to ensure that patients receive safe, effective care. The responsibilities of the first line nurse manager (Head nurse) toward staff include:

1. Staff utilization
2. Staff supervision
3. Staff development
4. Staff evaluation.

Staff utilization

- Assign tasks to staff members. Each staff member knows to whom he/she is responsible, who is responsible to him/her and for what. Authority must accompany responsibility for the staff nurse in order to carry out the assigned tasks. Conformity with hospital policies is essential.
- Plan time schedule of staff in advance taking into account personal requests and maintain.
- An effective means of communication, e.g. planned and incidental conferences, written reports, records, etc.
- An environment free from distracters and conducive to better performance.

Staff supervision

- Establish a harmonious relationship with staff.
- Inform the staff what you expect of them and make it clear that what kind of performance is anticipated from them.

Staff development

Help the staff members to develop their highest potential.

- Involve staff members in developing their knowledge and skills and positive attitudes for patient care and in establishing objectives and criteria for their attainment.
- Encourage staff to participate in planning for the improvement of nursing care and to apply research findings, case presentations, attending work shops and conferences, etc.

Staff evaluation

- Evaluate staff performance objectively by monitoring and maintaining a routine system for their continuous evaluation and ensure the attainment of objectives.
- Encourage the staff to evaluate their own work, analyze problems and decides on actions to resolve problems. Self-evaluation helps the individual to determine her/his progress and assist her/him for continuous growth.
- Investigate any complaints or lack of cooperation between nursing staff and help establish a pleasant atmosphere on the unit.

Nursing Unit Management

Maintain smooth coordination and relationship with in the department (intra-departmental) and with other departments (inter-departmental) that relate directly or indirectly to patient care.

Main functions of head nurse

Admissions and discharges:

Management of patient admissions: Greet new patient, introduce self and others.

Orientation of patients to services of the unit. Policies, rules, regulation, visiting hrs, food timings, etc.

Management of patient discharge: Give all instructions for follow-up care; inform family, hand over belongings.

Doctor's rounds: Activities to be performed before rounds:
- To keep ready all investigations.
- To complete patient charts organized, in order and ready.
- To keep unit ready.
- All equipment in order.
- All the patients are in bed.

Activities during Doctor's rounds
- Assist with the examinations
- Take notes on significant comments
- Report symptoms, reactions, etc.

Activities after rounds:
- See that the patients are comfortable.
- Carry out the changes ordered, e.g. investigations, new medication, stat orders, etc.

Drug administration: Check for drug stocks, narcotics and drugs nearing expiry date and take necessary action.

Operation theatre administration (OR): Check OR list, patient and family is informed, preoperative preparation, patient consent and chart is complete, etc.

Inter departmental coordination: Establish good interpersonal relationship with other health service departments in the hospital and ensure effective coordination to improve patient care.

For example: dietary, laundry, laboratory, X-ray, blood bank, general services, biomedical engineering deptt., etc.

Reporting:
- Make daily written report of problems of patient care and unit management to the supervisor or the director of nursing service (Nursing officer) at the end of the shift.
- Maintain incident reports of any untoward happenings.

MANAGEMENT STANDARDS

Objectives

1. Explain each of the nursing service standards.
2. Describe the relationship between standards of nursing service and their management implications.

JCAH (Joint Commission of American Hospital) NURSING SERVICES STANDARDS

Standards	Emphasis
Standard I	The nursing department/service shall be directed by a qualified nurse administer and shall be appropriately integrated with the medical staff and with other hospital staffs that provide and contribute to patient care. The administrator of the nursing department/service shall be a qualified, Registered nurse with appropriate education, experience, and licensure and demonstrated ability in nursing practice and administration.
Standard II	The nursing department/service shall be organized to meet the nursing care needs of patients and to maintain established standards of nursing practice. The nursing department/service shall have a written organizational plan that delineates lines of authority, accountability and communication. The manner in which the nursing department/service is organized shall be consistent with the variety of patient services offered and the scope of nursing care activities. Reviewing and approving policies and procedures. Establishing standards of nursing care accounting for professional and administrative nursing staff activities. Implementing the approved policies of the nursing department/service. Appointing committees as needed. Encouraging nursing staff personnel to participate in staff education programs.
Standard III	Nursing department/service assignments in the provision of nursing care shall be commensurate with the qualifications of nursing personnel and shall be designed to meet the nursing care needs of patient. A sufficient number of qualified registered nurses shall be on duty at all times to give patients the nursing care that requires the judgment and specialized skills of a registered nurse.
Standard IV	Individualized, goal-directed nursing care shall be provided to patients through the use of the nursing process. The nursing process (assessment, planning, intervention, evaluation) shall be documented for each hospitalized patient from admission through discharge.
Standard V	Nursing department/service personnel shall be prepared through appropriate education and training programs for their responsibilities in the provision of nursing care. Education/training programs for nursing department/service personnel shall be ongoing and designed to augment their knowledge of pertinent new developments in patient care and to maintain current competence. The scope and complexity of program shall be based on the documented educational needs of nursing staff personnel and the resources available to meet those needs.
Standard VI	Written policies and procedures that reflect optimal standards of nursing shall guide the provision of nursing care.

Written standards of nursing practice and reflected policies and procedures shall define and describe the scope and conduct of patient care provided by the nursing staff. These standards, policies and procedures shall be reviewed at least annually, revised as necessary, dated to indicate the time of the last review, signed by the responsible reviewing authority and implicated.

Standard VII As part of the hospitals quality assurance program, the quality and appropriateness of the patient care provided by the nursing department/service are monitored and evaluated and identified problems are resolved.

The nursing department/service has a planned and systematic process for monitoring and evaluation of the quality and appropriateness of patient care and for resolving identified problems.

Every institution/health care agency need to develop their own standards for providing quality patient care as per the international standards set for the nursing practice.

Unit VII: Personnel Management—Directing

16 Staffing

OBJECTIVES

1. Discuss the staffing process in a health agency.
2. Analyze factors that affect staffing in a given unit.
3. Calculate the staffing need in a nursing unit.
4. Analyze the importance of job description.

INTRODUCTION

Staffing is an orderly, systematic process based upon sound rationale applied to determine.
- The number and kind of nursing personnel required to provide nursing care of predetermined standard to group of patients in a particular setting.

The End Result

Prediction of the kind and number of staff to give care to patients. Staffing is to determine how many people of what specific skills are needed when they are needed, and ensuring their availability.

OBJECTIVES OF STAFFING

- To provide qualified nursing personnel in sufficient number.
- To ensure adequate, safe nursing care for all patients 24 hrs a day, 7 days a week, and 52 weeks a year.

FACTORS WHICH AFFECT STAFFING

1. Philosophy and objectives of the agency
2. Factors related to clients
3. Factors related to personnel
4. Factors related to work environment

Philosophy and Objectives

Philosophy and objectives of an organization should guide staffing pattern. Clearly defined objectives will help in planning the staff required to provide patient care adequately and assures quality care.

Client Factors

The type of patients or category of patients admitted to the hospital or health care agency. Acuity levels which refers to the functional ability of the patients, fluctuation in admissions, length of stay in the hospital, type of care required for each category of patients, and standards of nursing care to be met.

Personnel Factors

The staffing factors which include the employee's category, educational and experience levels of staff, job descriptions, mix of levels and titles, absenteeism, and personnel polices such as holidays week ends, sick leave, over time and the market.

Work Environment Factors

The organizational structure, type of support services and personnel, number of beds, general supplies and equipment, nurse-patient ratio required (1:1 in critical care) and the budget.

Every factor has its own strength and weakness and affects staffing which reflects on the quality ultimately.

Staffing Process

Staffing is a logical operation that consists of several independent actions.
1. Identify the type and amount of nursing care needed by the patient.
2. Determine personnel categories that have the knowledge and skills to perform needed care measures.
3. Predicting the number of personnel in each job category that will be need to meet anticipated care demands.
4. Obtaining budgeted positions for the number in each job category needed to care for the expected types and number of patients.
5. Recruiting personnel to fill available applicants.
6. Selecting and appointing personnel from available applications.
7. Combining personnel into desired configuration, by unit and shift.
8. Orienting personnel to fulfill assigned responsibilities.
9. Assigned responsibilities for patient care to available personnel.

Patient Care Needs

The nurse manager must be aware of the total number of patients on the ward to be cared for and the proportion in each category such as self care, minimal care, full care, and intensive care because nursing care needs vary from one category to an other. In order to quantify nursing work load patient care needs must be quantified.

Total care needs for each patient are the sum of the patient's needs for direct care and indirect care.

Direct Patient Care × Indirect Care = Total Patient Care Needs

Direct care: It is the care given by nursing personnel while working in the presence of patient and related to the patient physical and psychological needs.

Direct care involves; feeding, hygiene, treatment, mobility and the medication, etc. The more dependent the patient is on the nurse to carry out related activity, the more hours of nursing care is needed for that patient.

Indirect care: Indirect care are those activities undertaken on the patient behalf away from his presence.

Activities of indirect care include assembling supplies and equipment, consulting with other health care team members, writing and reading patient records, reporting, preparing discharge plans, preparation and cleaning up required equipment before and after procedures, etc. Generally, a patient indirect care needs do not vary with the intensity of illness or dependency and assumed to require the same amount of time for all patients in the unit.

Example: 40 minutes/patient/day

When making plans for staffing, the manager must utilize and interpret the statistics. Based on the statistics of anticipated daily average patient census, seasonal variations, type of patients admitted, acuity of illness may be forecasted. Staffing needs usually projected for the fiscal year ahead. For scheduling reasons the need could be projected on daily basis utilizing patient classification system.

Time Standard

- It is to distinguish a value of unit (usually a measure of time) to various activities of patient care. Those activities are usually clustered according to the above mentioned categories such as feeding, hygiene, etc.
- When figuring time standards for nursing care, one should consider both direct and indirect care. Once the number and kind of care activities required for each patient are identified then the length of time it takes to do the activities calculated.
- One can add up the time required by all patients on the ward or unit and divide by the number of productive work hours on a shift for one nurse to determine the number of personnel needed.
- The mix of nursing personnel can be predicted by categorizing the care needed by the qualification to give it.
- Adding the time in each category, dividing by productive hours on a shift, and obtaining the number of specific types of personnel required to meet the patient's needs.

Calculation of the Required Number of Staffing

Identify the nursing care hours required to care for each patient for a day or for a shift.

If patient categories are considered, then estimate the total care hours required for each patient in each category including both direct and indirect care hours. Nursing care hours are identified by deciding on the nursing care activities needed to care for each patient depending on the level of care required, identifying the frequency of those activities and the average time required to perform each activity, multiplying the average time by the related frequency, and total up to get an estimate of nursing care hours needed for a patient. After estimating the nursing care hours required, you could apply the following formula to estimate the number of nurses needed.

Nursing care hours required × average patient census × 365 = (365 – expected days off for one nurse) × number of work hours of one nurse per day.

The result of this equation is the number of nurses needed for the fiscal year.

The same equation can be used to calculate the number needed for each shift or for the whole day, or for one year, for each category of patients, or to decide the mix from each category of nursing, just by calculating the related required hours.

Example: If you want to identify only the number needed for one shift; identify care hours needed for that shift for a patient, multiply by the average census, and divide by work hours of one nurse in that shift.

Formula:

$$\frac{\text{Care hrs needed per patient per shift} \times \text{average census}}{\text{Work hrs of one nurse in that shift}}$$

PRACTICAL EXERCISE

Assume that you are working as head nurse in a medical ward.
- Identify the process of staffing and estimate the required number of nurses for the year and for the shift in your unit.
- Estimate following the method discussed above, the number of nurses needed for your unit for an year and for a shift.
- Identify the factors you considered in deciding the number of staff.

17. Scheduling/Duty Roster

OBJECTIVES

1. Describe the concept, purposes and principles of time planning (Duty Roster)
2. Explain the importance scheduling and scheduling policies.
3. Identify steps used in planning duty roster.
4. Discuss the guide lines followed in preparing the duty roster.

INTRODUCTION

In nursing management of any unit, time planning for the workers is a pre-requisite for successful nursing operations, because patterning of working and non-working hours directly affect the employee's productivity, work satisfaction and job tenure.

So, scheduling is defined as a patterns of on-off duty hours for employees in a particular unit.

Purposes of Scheduling

1. To ensure adequate patient care while over staffing is avoided.
2. To achieve desirable distribution of days off.
3. To ensure faire treatment of nursing staff.
4. To let individuals know in advance what their schedules are.
5. To achieve good unit management.
6. To determine when the help is required from the relief nurse.

Principles in Planning the Duty Roster (Fig. 17.1)

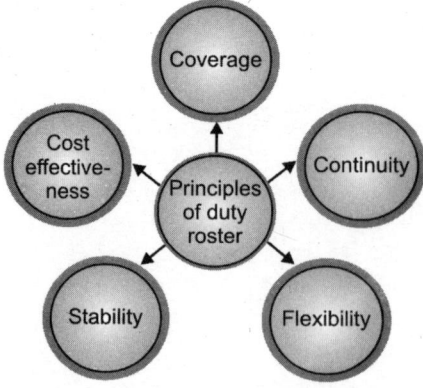

Fig. 17.1: Principles of duty roster

1. **Coverage:** Nursing coverage must be provided 24 hrs a day, seven days a week with the right number and mix of the staff.
2. **Continuity:** Continuity of quality and quantity of care.
3. **Flexibility:** The ability of the scheduling system to handle change and consider individual preferences as much as possible.
4. **Stability:** The extent to which nurses know in advance their future days off and on duty and in consistent with stable staffing policies.
5. **Cost effectiveness:** The ability to assign the needed staff without over staff and ensuring maximum utilization of nurse's time and skills.

Scheduling Policies

There should be department policies to guide managers in distributing desirable and undesirable work hrs equitably among employees.

Some Example of Policies

- A policy for a person, by title, who is responsible for preparing the roster.
- The time period to be covered by each schedule.
- The number of weeks or days in advance that the roster should be posted.
- The total of on duty hours for each employee.
- The beginning and ending hours of each shift, break times.
- Number of shifts to which each employee must rotate, days off, week ends offs per month, minimum days off in sequence.
- Number of paid holidays and vacation days, vacation scheduling.
- Procedure for handling emergency requests, number of sequential work days.
- Shift pattern (8 hrs, 10 hrs, and 12 hrs shifts) with different combination of working days and off days.

Steps in Planning Duty Roster

1. A skeleton plan is made in pencil to allow alterations.
2. The general steps that may be taken when building up the plan are.
3. List the names in order of seniority.
4. Put special requests in ink to avoid erasure.
5. Insert days off, noting busier days. It is important not to have too many nurses off duty at the same time.
6. When placing in days off in the schedule, refer to previous roster so that days offs are reasonably spaced and weekend offs are shared.
7. Add the shifts, balancing senior and junior nurses on each shift, ensuring that there is a senior nurse on duty to take charge, and that the trained nurses are evenly distributed.
8. Total the number of staff on duty for each shift.
9. Roster may be planned weekly or monthly or may be a fixed one.
10. All the above mentioned steps can be modified based on the policies of each organization to suit the working conditions.

Holidays

The charge nurse should be aware of the holiday allotted to each of the staff nurse, who should also be fully aware of her holidays allotted to her.

Nurses should be encouraged to plan their holidays a head of time.

Only certain number of staff should be allowed to take their holiday's. At the same time the number is usually agreed between the charge nurse and the nurse administrator.

Guide to Compiling Duty Roster (PART A)

1. Use roster sheet as provided by health agencies.
2. Do not cut sheets-always use full size and fill one sheet before going on to new sheet.
3. Compile roster for one full calendar month in advance.
4. Fill in headings-name of department-month dates and days of week.
5. Rule lines in Red to divide into complete weeks, e. g. from Saturday of the previous week to Friday of the following week.
6. Write Full Name and designation of each staff member in left hand column.
7. Ensure that the names of all staff including those on leave and new members are recorded accurately.
8. When staff leave the department through transfer or resignation, draw two lines in red through remaining days of the month, indicating the new department, or resignation, or end of contract.
9. Enter leave by ruling a line between the agreed dates. For example, _____ 30 days AL + 45 days ML – 15.12.2007 _____
10. Use accepted symbols only:

Symbols:		
AL	-	Annual Leave.
ML	-	Maternity Leave.
SL	-	Sick Leave.
AWOL	-	Absent without Leave.
Sty. L	-	Study Leave.
N/O	-	Nursing Officer.
NS	-	Nursing Super in Tendeut
Wd/N	-	Ward Nurse.
HN	-	Head Nurse.
Dy. W/N	-	Deputy Ward Nurse.
N/SPVR	-	Nurse Supervisor.
Sen. S/N	-	Senior Staff Nurse.
S/N	-	Staff Nurse.
A/N	-	Assistant Nurse.
M/O	-	Medical Orderly.
St. N	-	Student Nurse.

Guide to compiling Duty Roster (Part B)

1. Before starting, check request book for any special requests.
2. All shifts M (morning), A (afternoon), N (night) should be written in blue felt pen.
3. DO (day off), PH (public health holiday) should be written in top right corner, e.g. PH^6, etc.
4. Asterisk (*) the name of the staff nurse in charge for each shift.
5. Count numbers on each shift according to grade, total and record on roster.
6. Duty roster should be submitted to nursing officer NS for checking and approval one week before they are due to come into force.
7. Staff who resigns at any time during the year are only entitled to the number of PHs occurring up to the date of resignation.
8. Copy of the completed roster checked and signed by the ward incharge and nursing officer is to be submitted to nursing administration not later than 26th/27th day of each month.

18 Job Description

OBJECTIVES

1. Discuss the duties and responsibilities of a specific job.
2. Explain the information included in the job description.
3. Describe the purposes of job description.
4. Identify the guide lines for writing job description.

INTRODUCTION

In any organization the individuals working in a specific field need to understand what is expected of them by an health care agency. It is the responsibility of the management to write down the specific job functions according to the assignment given to the individual worker at the time of recruitment and make it clear to the employee. So that the worker will know the DOS and DONTS of his responsibilities as per the policies laid down by the management.

DEFINITION OF JOB DESCRIPTION

It refers to the duties and responsibilities of a specific job and the characteristics of the individual needed to perform it successfully.

It is a primary management vehicle for communicating the duties, responsibilities, scope of authority, organizational relationship, and personnel qualification for each job in the organization.

The duties listed in the job description should encompass all of what the employee is expected to do during normal work week, plus some duties regularly recurring every two or four weeks, if known.

As long as the basic list of duties encompass 90–95% of employees work, sufficient for performance appraisal.

Information Included in the Job Description

Information included in the job description may vary from one organization to another but would include the following.

1. Job title
2. Department
3. Job grade
4. The date of the job description; besides the duties and responsibilities.

Example

Job Description

1. Job title: Nursing director
2. Department: Nursing services of KC General hospital
3. Job grade: Special Grade I
4. The date of the job description : 10.10.07
5. Accountability: To whom the employee is accountable to report and under whose direction he/she is expected to carry out the duties assigned.

Purposes of Preparing Job Description in the Organization

Job descriptions are used for:

1. Job analysis and classification
2. Recruitment
3. Delegation of responsibilities
4. Staff development
5. Staff appraisal

Guidelines for writing job description:

1. Allocate a title that distinctively implies the nature of a job.
2. Introduce the description with a summary of the essential features of a particular job.
3. Organize the list of requirements and duties in a logical sequence, concentrating on the major work activities and the proportion of time involved.
4. Write in a clear, concise manner, avoiding ambiguity and too much detail.
5. Use standard formats for all job descriptions.
6. Review periodically.

19 Performance Appraisal

OBJECTIVES

1. Describe the concept and objectives of staff evaluation.
2. Discuss the qualities to be evaluated.
3. Explain and discuss the staff evaluation tools and techniques and the characteristics of an effective evaluation tool.
4. Discuss the appraisal interview and evaluation report.

INTRODUCTION

An organization must evaluate the performance status of its staff if it is to proper, since all organizational achievements are dependent upon its human resources. Meanwhile, the staff in the organization needs feedback concerning their personal accomplishment. Staff evaluation is a continuous process and it starts with the first contact with the time the person is employed and ends with his retirement.

Employee performance is the product of: ability, motivation, and environment, and the performance appraisal system addresses only the first two. Accurate appraisal is an effective means for increasing productivity, and people learn best when they receive immediate feedback. Who should evaluate? The direct supervisor, so it's the in-charge nurses responsibility to evaluate all nurses working in the unit with her, and to evaluate correctly she should be in frequent, direct and prolonged contact, so she can observe an adequate sample of all aspects of nurses performance. When evaluation takes place? Informal evaluation and feedback should be done on continuous bases, but the formal evaluation is done every six months or at the end of the year, and at the end of probation period.

DEFINITION

A periodic formal evaluation of how well personnel have performed their duties during a specific period, it is a systematic, interpersonal, continuous process between manager, and employee involving job guidelines and objectives and job descriptions.

Objectives

1. To determine job competence.
2. To select qualified individuals for promotion or transfer.
3. To establish and improve:
   - Communication between supervisors and subordinates.
   - Staff performance.

4. To determine:
   - Training and developmental needs of staff.
   - Salary standards and to award merit.
5. To provide the staff with recognition for accomplishment.
6. To discover the aspirations and talents of the staff.
7. To check the efficacy of staff development programs.
8. To identify unsatisfactory staff for demotion or termination.
9. To aid the manager in coaching and counseling.

Principles of Evaluation

First, the employees evaluation should be based on behaviorally stated performance standards, which should be reflected in the job description and related performance standards, and the employees should be aware of them as their desirable performance goals.

Second, an adequate representative sample of the nurse's job should be observed to provide the basis of evaluation.

Third, the nurse should be given a copy of job description, performance standards, and performance evaluation form, to understand how she was evaluated.

Fourth, when documenting the evaluation, the manager should indicate the satisfactory and unsatisfactory areas of performance.

Fifth, areas of performance that need improvement should be stated according to priority.

Sixth, the evaluation interview should be scheduled in proper time and environment.

Seventh, the goal of evaluation should improve performance and satisfaction, rather than punish.

Qualities to be Evaluated

Since, evaluation will be made by various individuals; if necessary to define carefully each quality should be evaluated. The qualities most frequently evaluated fall under five major headings:

1. **Quality of performance,** i.e. the evaluation of both the quantity and quality of work, neatness, orderliness, reliability, accuracy, knowledge of work, execution, etc.
2. **Mental qualities,** i.e. the ability to learn, adaptability, reasoning power, judgment, memory, etc.
3. **Supervisory qualities,** i.e. leadership and organizational ability, communication skill cooperation, etc.
4. **Personnel qualities,** i.e. honesty, self-control, self-confidence, initiative, attitude towards others, team work, appearance, etc.
5. **Capacity of further development,** i.e. intelligence, acceptance of responsibility and other features inherent in leadership.

Problems in Performance Appraisal

Halo effect, is the tendency to overrate a person because of his pleasant personality, strong social skills, he performed well in past, recent good performance not the whole year, or share the interests of the manager.

Horn effect, is the tendency to rate employees lower than what he deserves because: she/he committed a serious error recently, disagrees with the manager, fails to meet manager standards for dress and behavior, or poor performing peers.

The central tendency error, is the tendency to rate the employee in the middle of the range for each dimension.

Self aggregating effect, when the manager deliberately crafts ratings to create an image of their own leadership style.

Staff Evaluation Tools and Techniques

Tools and techniques are used to compare output (staff performance) to goals (Job description and individual goals).

The Characteristics of Evaluation Tool

An evaluation tool, to be an effective, should be designed to reduce bias, increase objectivity and ensure validity and reliability.
1. **Objectivity** is the ability to remove oneself emotionally from a situation so as to consider the facts without distortion by personnel feelings.
2. **Validity** is the degree to which a tool measures what it intends to measure.
3. **Reliability** concerns consistency of results, that is whether several raters using the same tool to rate an employee produce the same or similar ratings or results. This is called the inter-rater reliability.

Another reliability measure, intra-rater reliability, is whether the same rater rates an employee with the same or similar results on two or more different occasions, assuming that the employee's performance has not changed. Reliability is important because a tool must be reliable before it can be valid.

The most commonly used evaluation tools are:

1. **Rating scale:** The most common only used tool in nursing service. It consists of set of behaviors or characteristics to be rated and same types of scales for indicating the degree to which each present. The scale my take several forms, numerical, graphic or descriptive.
2. **Faced choice rating:** The technique requires the rater to select from groups of statements that best fit and least the individuals being rated. The statement are in behavioral terms and are weighed and scored.
3. **Check-list:** It is compressed of a series of descriptive statement in behavioral terms about the standard of nursing performance of the job expected of the individual nurse. The rater places a mark in the "yes" or "no" column in accordance with individual's behavior. A space is provided for those item which are not applicable

the items are weighed in pre-established values to secure total rating this tool is easier and tend to reduce bias but it needs time and effort to develop a valid check-list tool. The check-list is an efficient tool of assessing technical procedures and in handling large number of staff.
4. **Critical incident technique:** Anecdotal record in this technique, the rater records of positive and negative behaviors considered critical to the employee's success on the job behaviors are recorded, not the manager's interpretation or judgment of the behavior.

    Critical incidents should be related of the job duties and responsibilities or to individual goals the following is an example related to a job duty of a staff nurse. That is formulating and recording appropriate nursing care plan for assigned patients.
5. **Management by objective (MBO):** The nurse manager (rater) evaluates the staff according to predetermined goals or objective that have been jointly arrived at by her/him and the individual staff. Comparing staff the output to goals is an inherent part of the MBO concept. In MBO the source from which behaviors are to be rated. Come from individual employee's goals while the source of the others tools is the job description of the individual staff.

    Example for each patient to whom I am assigned, I will establish a nursing diagnosis write short-range goals to guide nursing care construct a written plan for nursing care.
6. **Peer-review:** In this method, the individual staff evaluated at the same time by the immediate supervisor plus three or four other supervisors, who have knowledge of that individual work performance the virtue of this method is it's thoroughness it is possible for multiple raters to modify or cancel out bias displayed by the immediate supervisor.

    Peer review is based on appraisal tools, these tools may address technical competence, human relation, communication, organizational, leadership and other skills the process must be determined and staff must be oriented to the system. Peer review could also include self evaluation.
7. **The state nursing competencies rating scale:** The scale measures the competencies displayed by a nurse so as she/he performs nursing actions.

    Example gives explains and verbal reassurance when needed.
8. **The essay:** The rater writes one or more paragraph about how well the employee performs and his or her strength and weaknesses in relations to the tasks identified in the job description this method needs time and efforts. On the other hand, it can give data about an employee's developmental needs.

The Appraisal Interview

The objective of a personal interview in to evaluate past, present, and future potential of an individual.

The following points are general guidelines for the nurse manager:
1. Establish a friendly atmosphere by selecting the right time and place for the interview. Be sure the interview will be free of interruptions.
2. Ensure freedom from work assignment. Arrange for coverage during the time of meeting. Begin and end the session on time.
3. Establish rapport - a few brief chit-chat before the actual interview.
4. Let the individual talk first. Include all important issues in the discussion. Be alert present criticism carefully. Never combine positive and negative comments and use the guidance approach. Use a concerned tone of voice. Discuss the work never the worker.
5. Make a final overall judgment about the individual progress, as well as any recommendations on the evaluations form.
6. Let the individual sign the report and explain that the signatures does not necessarily signify that she/he agrees with content, but it indicates that she/he has seen it.
7. Prepare a list of objective for modifying or improving behaviors for the next operational period.
8. Never create a threatening or bargaining environment.

Evaluation Report

The evaluation report is to be written jointly by the nurse manager and staff nurse. It should be reliable, valid and accurate, showing progress made by the staff nurse and giving illustrations to substantiate value judgments. If both have kept notes that they have periodically assessed and if the staff nurse believes the nurse manger's intent is to help rather than to blame, the staff nurse will feel more free to be honest in an evaluation of her/his strengths and weaknesses. If the staff nurse has not been functioning satisfactorily, she/he will already be aware of it. If her/his performance has not improved adequately since previous interviews, the staff nurse should be informed that the weakness will be included in the report. Any improvements are to be noted, and the staff nurse should know exactly where she/he stands. It may be necessary to tell her/him that she/he has to make certain improvements within a definite time period.

20 Staff Motivation

OBJECTIVES
- Describe the need for motivation and the concept of motivation.
- Discuss the theories of motivation.
- Describe the measures taken by the nurse manager to facilitate nurses' motivation.

INTRODUCTION
An important function of the nurse manager is to motivate nursing staff on the job produce high quantity and high quality of work. To do that is not a simple task, and there are no simple rules that the manger could follow to stimulate the staff, but there are different theories that suggest answers to, why do people work; why do some people achieve high productivity level, and what can a manger do to stimulate intrinsic and extrinsic motivation.

DEFINITION
Motivation is "an inner impulse or an internal force that initiates and directs the individual to act in a certain manner to satisfy a need."

Motivating force is a need that comes from within an individual, e.g. to make a living, gain status and respect or to remove a source of frustration (Review of Maslow's Hierarchy of Needs).

Motivation is a process which begins with a need that must be satisfied by the individual who feels it. This results in a activity and or behavior that is intended to satisfy the need. If activity or behavior is blocked, it results in frustration.

NEED FOR MOTIVATION
The nurse manager must realize that nurses have different personalities, work habits, and what motivates one nurse may not motivate others. Meanwhile, some nurses are skilled, confident, and capable of self-direction and seem to motivate themselves, while other nurses lack self-confidence; they do their jobs poorly and have little motivation. The nurse manager is responsible to motivate the second group and to improve their performance.

Researches have revealed that job performance is the result of the interaction of two variables; the ability to perform the task and the amount of motivation.

Job Performance = Ability + Motivation.

Job Dissatisfaction

Job dissatisfaction contributes to higher turnover rates and decreased productivity and considerable time and money are required to recruit and select a replacement for some one who leaves the organization, it also takes time to socialize new employee to the organizational culture, which is expensive time, beside that, other employees will need to carry more load to cover the needs, and at last the kind of interruptions that results from the loss of this employee. For all those reasons the manager should be concerned about job satisfaction of employee, and to do that there is a need to look at the different theories.

Motivation Theories

Taylor's Monistic theory, Taylor believed that if energetic people with high productivity learned that they earned no more than a lazy worker, he would lose interest in hard work, and incentive system is needed to prevent this loss, so it should be possible to earn more by producing more. In contrast to Taylor's belief that money is a primary motivator, Maslow maintained that people are motivated by the desire to satisfy a hierarchy of needs, and the satisfaction of one level triggers the emergence of higher needs and that a satisfied need is no longer a motivator, according to his Hierarchy of needs theory.

According to McClelland's basic needs theory, all people have three basic needs in varying degree; the need for achievement, power and affiliation. People with high achievement needs are eager for responsibility, take risks and desire feedback. People with high affiliation need seek meaningful relationships and they want to be respected by colleagues and avoid decisions or actions that oppose group norms. Managers should match personnel needs with assignments.

Argyris in his psychological energy theory believes that people will exert more energy to meet their own needs than those of the organization and the greater the disparity between the tow, the more likely it is that the employee will feel dissatisfaction, tension, conflict or apathy, he suggests that managers should match personnel and jobs taking into consideration their talents and interests, and help them satisfy their needs together with the organizational needs.

Vroom in his expectancy theory states that motivation is dependent on how much people want something and their estimate of the probability of getting it if they exert certain effort. So to be highly motivated, a person needs to find an outcome attractive, believe that certain actions will lead to the desired outcome, and assess that the result is worth the effort. Consequently to motivate personnel the manager should clarify the connection between work and outcome.
(Herzberg's motivation – Hygiene theory)

It is important for the nurse manager to understand what encourages individuals to apply their ability and energy at work, the best motivator according to Herzberg is a challenging job that allows a feeling of achievement, earned recognition, enjoyment of the work itself. (Job content), suitable responsibility, job advancement, the possibility of growth (self-improvement).

It is also important for the nurse manager to understand what discourages individuals and makes them dissatisfied at work. They are:

Inefficient manager, Incompetent supervision, Poor interpersonal relations, Personal qualities of the manager, Inadequate pay, Improper working conditions like heat, dust and noise, Timings and long working hours, Inadequate pay, Improper working conditions like heat, dust and noise, timings and long working hours, Inadequate and nonfunctioning equipment.

One of the great challenges in motivation is manager's ability to help their subordinates really understand their needs and satisfy them.

MEASURES TAKEN BY THE NURSE MANAGER TO FACILITATE NURSES MOTIVATION

The nurse manager while managing the nursing unit will have to choose a combination of the following measures to facilitate nurses' motivation.

Act as a Role model (Set a good example):
- Set high standards in the units.
- Maintain a positive attitude towards the work and staff.
- Be optimistic; in other words, be aware of how difficult the job is and how it can be done.
- Ask for help when in need.
- Admit mistakes.
- Develop and maintain Good Personal Relations
- Use two-way communication.
- Be friendly, not to criticize staff in front of others and be fair.
- Keep a sense of humor and avoid getting angry.
- Try to understand nurses' attitudes, likes, dislike their experience, previous training, problems in their work and needs.

These measures will help in understanding nurses' behavior. Understanding is the first step toward motivating nurses. Trust comes with understanding and it develops slowly based on the respect and acceptance of the manager. Motivation is based on understanding and trust.

Some Guidelines for Developing Trust

- Apply rules equally and consistently.
- Avoid favoring some nurses over others, be fair.
- Share information – show respect for ideas and opinions and confidentiality.
- Be supportive at all times.

Post each nurse where she can work best

The nurse is more likely to succeed and be motivated if her/his interests and skills are considered in the assignment. Success is the best motivator.

Use a Participative Style

Participation and sharing information will motivate nurses since they feel they are taking part in decisions. Motivation requires more than physical involvement in a job. It also demands mental and emotional involvement.

Guide, Encourage and Support Continuously

Guidance means helping nurses in planning, evaluating their work and in solving work and personal problems. Consider individual differences, be sensitive to variations in nurses' needs, abilities and goals, and provide realistic job information, clear instructions and feedback.

Encouragement means helping and reassuring nurses regardless of the type of problems. Develop a supportive environment by reducing physical stresses associated with the job. Encourage nurses to make decisions. Encourage skilled nurses to share their expertise with less experienced nurses so that both of them are motivated to continue their role.

Support means removing obstructions and providing nurses with satisfying work environment which include personnel and facilities and suitable learning materials needed to do their job. Also, improving job content to include more planning and self-direction.

Reward Good Work

Give recognition for successful achievement of the job. Praise frequently and informally. It can be in front of other staff.

Reward includes: Pay increase, promotion, training for advancement to a higher level within a job.

Thank you is a type of reward that helps to increase self-confidence.

Build team work (Team spirit)

Schedule Regular Meetings

- Make nurses feel that their job is important to the success of the team.
- Integrate the needs and wants of the staff nurses with those of the nursing unit.
- Think of nurses in the unit as a group and do what is best for them.

Provide Continuing Education

Nurses enjoy learning new knowledge and skills or updating the existing knowledge and skills or taking new responsibilities through continuing education.

SYMPTOMS OF MOTIVATED NURSES

- Show interest, enthusiasm and have a positive attitude.
- Believe their work is important and work hard.
- Work well with their supervisors and others.

- Take part willingly in planning, implementing and evaluating their work.
- Show responsible behavior.
- Strive to find the best way to produce optimal job performance.

Exercise

Topic: Quality assurance.

Purpose: The session will prepare students to:
- Understand quality assurance and infection control process and different related possible structures.
- Understand the importance of identifying and measuring quality indicators.
- Understand nursing standards: how they are developed, by whom, etc.

Directions: Divide the group 5-8 in each and assign each group to:
- Discuss as an individual or a group with the in-charge or the coordinator of the quality assurance and infection control system and the process in the nursing department, and related policies.
- Identify the quality indicators used in the unit and suggest other important indicators that could be used.
- Identity and discuss the nursing care standards used in the nursing department or unit and how they are developed and by whom.
- Get copies of different standards and incident form.
- During session, the groups.
- Participate in the discussion about quality assurance process.
- Proposes as a group a structure for QA for your hospital.
- Identity any ethical issue and develop scenario on it.
- Guidelines to the faculty.
- Prepare different groups with their discussions.
- Let the groups present and give feedback.
- Emphasize important policies related.
- Reinforce important points.

21

Staff Development

OBJECTIVES
- Discuss the concept and objectives of staff development.
- Discuss the types of staff development.

Explain the Staff Development Model

Describe the responsibility for conducting staff development programs and the role of the nurse manager in staff development.

STAFF DEVELOPMENT

Introduction

Staff development activities consist of the training and education provided by an employer to improve employee's occupational knowledge, skills and attitudes and to provide the employee with the opportunity to grow professionally.

Objectives
- To assist each employee to improve performance in present position.
- To keep in pace with medical sciences.
- New development in medical science and technology.
- New diagnostic and treatment techniques.
- To motivate each staff member and create a sense of security and loyalty.
- To improve work productivity and for promotion.
- To reduce staff turnover, absenteeism and tardiness.
- To acquire personal and professional abilities that maximize the possibility of career advancement.

Types

Staff development includes formal and informal, group or individual training and education.
 Staff development activities include:
1. Induction training,
2. Orientation,
3. In-service education,
4. Continuing education, and

5. Training for special functions such as management, team building, and budgeting method.

Induction Training (3 days): Is a brief introduction to agency philosophy, purpose, administrators, programs, policies and regulations that is given to new employee during the first three days of employment.

Orientation (2-24 weeks): Is individualized training given each employee during the first period of his job to familiarize him with his job's duties, work place, clients and coworker.

In-service education (2-8 hours): Includes all on-the-job instruction and training that is given to enhance employee's present job performance.

Continuing education (1-5 days): Includes all planned learning that is intended to increase employee's knowledge or skills beyond that needed for satisfactory performance in the present job.

For example: Training program at RUHSA.

STAFF DEVELOPMENT MODEL

The basic model of staff development process is similar to the nursing process and includes assessment, planning, implementation and evaluation (Fig. 21.1).

Assessment → Planning → Implementation → Evaluation

Fig. 21.1: Staff development model

Learner's readiness to learn	Finding resources	Learners	Cost effective achievement
Learning needs skill/ ability/knowledge	Matching needs and methods	Educators Materials Methods	Transfer of learning

Assessment is the process of investigation that provides knowledge about the learners' readiness to learn and learn and her or his specific learning needs, such as skill, ability or knowledge.

Planning is the process of obtaining learning resources to present to the learner and the matching of educational needs and methods.

Implementation is the gathering together of the customers, the learners and all of the materials and methods needed for the educational program(s) including the application of the Principles of Learning (Review Introduction to Teaching).

Evaluation is the investigative process in which to determine whether the education was cost-effective, the objectives were achieved and the learning was transferred from the learning site to actual use on the job.

EXAMPLE

Programs for Staff Development

Programs for staff development are developed around four areas of personnel needs.
- An introduction to their job (orientation).
- Training in both the manual and behavioral skills, associated with their jobs (skill training).
- Development of leadership and management abilities (Leadership and Management Development).
- Continuing investigation of the real potentialities of their job (Continuing Education).

Orientation Program

Definition: Orientation is the process of acquainting a new staff with the existing work environment so that he/she can relate quickly to his/her new surroundings.

Objective: To help new staff to adjust to new organization, environment, duties, etc. through a planned introduction of her/his responsibilities so that she/he can become efficient as soon as possible.

Orientation program is given at the initial stage of employment or when a staff takes on new responsibilities. It is designed to newly assigned staff. It consists of two parts: those instructions that must be given to any employee to be acquainted with overall purposes and functions and that relate to the specific job tasks that she/he must perform.

It is important that the new staff member does not assume full service responsibilities until orientation program has been carried through.

Advantages: Staff are helped to:
- Adjust to work situation.
- Be strongly motivated to learn.
- Be able to function effectively much sooner.
- Feel wanted and needed by coworkers and superiors.

Suggested content outline for an orientation program to the new nursing staff

1. *Environment and Personnel:* Orientation to environment, i.e. community setting served, hospital, nursing unit, residence and personnel such as administrative staff and workers, etc.
2. *Job Relationship:* Relationship of new nursing staff to other personnel, i.e. Nursing director, supervisor, head nurse, physiotherapist, social workers, etc. In other words, communication channels.
3. *Operational Policies:* Personal policies which affect the new staff, overall hospital policies and routines, physical set-up, philosophy and its relation to community.
4. *Services:* Nursing service department policies and unit and routines, i.e. hours of work, rotations, salaries, new methods and techniques used according to scientific advances, etc.

5. *Functions:* Employees job functions and responsibilities which may be assumed by the staff member and those of others, with whom she/he will be working (Job description).
6. *The Staff as an Individual:* Creation of a sense of need and interest in staff.
7. Relationship of the new nursing staff member to patients and their families.
8. Personal hygiene and maintenance of normal body functions.
9. Response of patients and their families to illness.
10. Human relationships in the hospital environment and their effects on a patient's response to illness and therapy.

In Large Institutions

It is practical to have all newly appointed nursing staff begin their work on the same day.

Group instructions can be arranged since several items on the orientation program are applicable to all categories of workers.

A more experienced nursing staff member is assigned as a preceptor to guide a newcomer, who can turn to her/him for any additional help and guidance she/he might need.

Skill Training Program

Objectives

To provide the nursing staff with the skills and attitudes required for the job and to keep them abreast of changing methods and new techniques.

Skill training may be manual or technical skills of doing for people (how and why) or skill in dealing and working well with people, patients as well as coworkers and accepting their behavioral patterns (human relations skill).

Skill training program is often a continuation of the orientation program. It is designed to new and older staff.

The following is a list of the key behaviors for skills training which include the "basic three" behaviors that should be followed for effective education.
- Presentation of the skill.
- Allowing the nursing staff to practice the skill.
- Providing feedback about that practice.

These behaviors incorporate most of the Principles of Learning.

Key Behaviors

- In writing, outline each step of the task to be taught.
- Explain the objectives of the task to the nursing staff.
- Show the nursing staff how to do it (without talking).
- Explain key points (Write them down if the are complex).
- Let the nursing staff watch you do it again.
- Let the nursing staff do the simple parts of the task (optional).

- Help the nursing staff do the whole task (watch and give feedback).
- Let the nursing staff do the whole task (give feedback when task is finished).
- Praise the nursing staff for doing the task correctly.

LEADERSHIP AND MANAGEMENT DEVELOPMENT

Objective

To improve managerial abilities of persons at every management level as well as potential managers to produce the greatest degree of organizational progress.

The proper approach to management development is a systems approach. The management development programs should be designed as an integrated whole, consisting of interrelated segments, each of which is devoted to one management function, i.e. planning, organizing, directing and controlling.

A management development program should begin by establishing agreement among top and middle level managers as to proper levels of authority, responsibility and accountability for managers at every level of the organizational hierarchy.

The need can be identified through the review of incident-reports, turnover rates, personnel and supply, costs per patient per day, patient audits or quality control reports.

Examples of topics for management development include: employment practices, types of leadership, decision-making, communication, performance appraisal, report writing, quality assurance, etc.

CONTINUING EDUCATION PROGRAM

Definition

Formal, organized, educational programs designed to promote the knowledge, skills and professional attitudes of nurses.

Objectives

To help the employee to:
- Keep up-to-date with new concepts and development in the health field.
- To increase their basis knowledge and skills and develop positive attitudes.
- Develop an ability to analyze problems and to work with others.
- Meet the challenge of changes in technology.
- Maintain standards of health care at acceptable level.
- Help in setting standards of performance.
- Improve understanding within the health care team.
- Help in career development.
- Motivate staff for better patient care.
- Meet new needs of the community.

Continuing education programs are usually short-term and specific, a certificate may be offered for completion of a course. It is not to be confused with academic, degree-granting programs such as advanced education or postgraduate education.

OTHER ACTIVITIES FOR STAFF DEVELOPMENT

The following are other activities which will stimulate the interest of the nursing staff to increase their knowledge and understandings and thus help them to develop (grow).

Attends conferences with the health team especially when one of her/his patients is being discussed.
1. Make rounds with the physicians.
2. Attend medical "ground round" in a teaching center.
3. Visit another hospital to observe their method of patient care.
4. Attend professional meetings, conferences, etc. and present papers.
5. Read articles of special interest and report them to staff.

THE RESPONSIBILITY FOR CONDUCTING STAFF DEVELOPMENT PROGRAMS

Most hospitals have a staff development coordinator who is responsible for chalking out continuing and in-service education programs. Also, staff nurses may be selected as preceptors to assist the new nurses in the unit based on their clinical competence, organizational skills, ability to guide and direct others. The preceptor's role is that of orienteer, teacher, resource person, counselor, role model and evaluator. Staff nurses (preceptors) benefit by having an opportunity to sharpen their clinical skills, increasing their personal and professional satisfaction. The education department assists the staff nurses.

THE ROLE OF THE NURSE MANAGER IN STAFF DEVELOPMENT

- Involves staff members in developing high standards of patient care and in establishing objectives and criteria for their attainment.
- Discover leadership's skills and creative abilities among staff and arrange for their development.
- Encourage staff to participate in planning for the improvement of nursing care and to apply findings of nursing practice research.
- Provide learning opportunities for professional advancement of staff in order to develop to their highest potential.
- Share in planning and participate in staff educational programs of professional and non-professional personnel.
- Allot time for discussions, observations and questions.
- Set a good example in everyday practice.

There should be written sources of information available for developing nursing staffing the hospital units in order to support learning. These are:
- Textbooks
- Procedure manuals
- Charts
- Periodicals
- Pamphlets
- Drug literature
- Equipment literature, etc.

Unit VIII: Controlling

22. Quality Assurance (QA)

OBJECTIVES

- Describe the concept of control in management process and specify its purposes and type.
- Specify the functions of nursing control system.
- Describe the concept and approaches to quality assurance.
- Discuss the steps of quality assurance process.
- Explain and discuss the quality assurance methods and the need for giving feedback to staff.

INTRODUCTION

Without a control system organizations have no indication of how well they perform in relation to their goals. Control provides an organization with a way to adjust its course if performance fails outside acceptable boundaries. Without effective control procedures, an organization is not likely to achieve its goals.

Controlling is essential in order to check, test regulate, verify and adjust. A prime element of the management of nursing services is a system for evaluation of the total effort.

This includes a system for evaluation of the management process as well as of the practice of Nursing. Evaluation requires standards than can be used as a yardstick for gauging the quality and the quantity of services.

DEFINITION

Controlling is regulation and monitoring of organizational activities in order to ensure compliance with standards set.

Purpose of Control

1. To detect deviations from desirable standards.
2. To take preventive and corrective actions in order to ensure that the organization's mission and objectives are accomplished as effectively and efficiently as possible.
3. To guide behavior and set in to motion plans for the future.

Types of Control

Anticipatory control: This addresses the question 'What can we do ahead of time to help our plan succeed.' Planned and preventive measures can save time, money, errors and legal problems.

For this, a manager needs to:
- Review mission and goals
- Review past success and failures
- Assess needs
- Project for the future

Concurrent Control

This type of control deals with present rather than the future or past. It involves monitoring and adjusting ongoing activities and processes to ensure compliance with standards. This occupies much of nurse manger's time because she is most concerned with the day-to-day activities of the unit.

For this a manager needs to:
- Monitor ongoing activities
- Make adjustments

Feedback Control

This involves gathering information about an ongoing or completed activity, evaluating that information and taking steps to improve that activity or similar activities in the future.

For this a manger needs to:
- Gather information on ongoing/completed activities.
- Learn from mistakes.
- Take steps to improve situation.

QUALITY ASSURANCE

The Joint Commission on the Accreditation of Health Care Organizations (JCAH), advocates that each hospital is required to conduct a comprehensive integrated Quality Assurance Program to ensure continuing control of quality care for patients.

The need for nursing quality assurance active is spelt out in the nursing standards of JCAH Manual. It states that "the Nursing Service Department" has a planned and systematic process for the monitoring and evaluation of the quality and appropriateness of patient care and for resolving identified problems. Nursing manager's understanding of the concept of quality assurance will enhance their role in implementing and evaluating standards of care.

Definition

Quality Assurance (QA) is the process of establishing a target degree of excellence for nursing intervention and taking action to ensure that each patient receives the agreed upon-level of care.

APPROACHES TO QUALITY ASSURANCE

There are three approaches from which nursing care can be evaluated to assure quality nursing practice:
- Structure,
- Process, and
- Outcome.

Since each of these interaction elements contributes to the quality of nursing care delivered, an improvement in any of the three tends to produce favorable change in the other two.

Structural Element

It includes the physical setting, instrumentality and conditions through which nursing care is administered, such as philosophy, objectives, policies, procedures, records, organizational structures, financial resources, equipment and expectations and attitudes of patients and employees.

Process Element

It includes steps of the nursing process itself – assessment, diagnosing, planning, implementation and evaluation and all subsystems within the nursing process, such as taking a health history, performing a physical examination, making a nursing diagnosis, determining nursing care goals, writing a nursing care plan, performing each care, cure and coordination of tasks prescribed by the care plan, measuring patient care outcome and recording and reporting patient's response to treatment. It is the criteria for measuring nursing care to determine if nursing standards of practice are being met, so they are task oriented.

Outcome Element

It includes changes in patient health systems that result from nursing interventions. Ex: modification in signs and symptoms, knowledge, attitudes satisfaction, skill level and compliance with treatment regimen, and established patient outcome criteria.

STEPS OF QUALITY ASSURANCE

QA is the systematic process of evaluating the quality of care given in a particular unit or institution. It involves the following steps:

Setting Standards

A standards is a desired quantity, quality or level of performance with reference to a criterion against which performance is to be measured. The nursing profession through the ANA itself has designated generic standards of nursing practice. In addition, each patient care unit must designated standards specific to the patient population served. These standards are the foundation upon which all other measures of QA are based.

For example: "Every patient will instruments are developed and selected to collect evidence that indicates standards are being met.

There are three basic forms of nursing audits: structure, process and outcome. Standards define nursing care customers as well as nursing activities of structural resources needed. They are used for planning nursing care as well as for evaluating it.

Assign Responsibility

Assign responsibility to individual or committee.

Delineate Scope of Care

Develop an inventory including the type of patients served, the conditions and diagnoses treated, the treatment or activities performed, the type of practitioners providing care, the site where care is provided. This will provide a bases for subsequent steps in the evaluation process.

Identify Important Aspects of Care

Unit personnel should ask themselves "which of the things we do are most important?" the answer should lead to identifying important aspects of care (criteria). Priority should be given to those aspects of care which occur frequently, affect large number of patients involves risk or serious consequences or will deprive patient from substantial benefit if the care is-not provided correctly or problematic behavior.

Determining Criteria

Criteria must be determined that will indicate if the standards are being met and to what degree they are met. Criteria must be general and specific to the individual unit. A criteria is the value-free name of a variable that is known to be reliable indicator of quality.

For example: A criterion to demonstrate that the standard regarding care plan for every patient is being met would be:

"A nursing care plan is developed and written by a registered nurse within 12 hours of admission." This criterion provides a measurable indicator to evaluate performance.

Data Collection

Sufficient observations and random samples are necessary for producing reliable and valid information. A useful rule is that 10 percent of the institutional patient population per month should be sampled.

Data collection methods include:
- Patients' observations and interviews.
- Nurses observations and interviews.
- Review of charts.

Evaluating Performance

The methods include:
- Reviewing documented records.
- Observing activities as they take place.
- Examining patients.
- Interviewing patients, families and staff.

Records are most commonly uses source for evaluation but they are not as reliable as direct observations. It is quite possible to write in the patient's chart activities that were not done or to not record these things that were done. Also, the chart indicates the care provided but it does not demonstrate the quality of that care.

For the stated criteria example: This step will be: Records would be examined to determine if care plans were written on each patient within 12 hours of admission and, if so, that standards had been met.

Another example: To measure quality of the care plan:

Every care plan will include patient education appropriate to the patient's medical diagnosis, nursing diagnosis, interventions planned and discharge planning.

Problem Identification

Analysis and reporting of the data gathered from the evaluation process will lead to problem identification and isolation and the evidence is gathered through round, observation and records. The nurse manager's responsibility is to look for patterns or trends of deviation from normal, further data collection and analysis could be done for the identified problems.

Problem Solution

Once problem has been defined and isolated, plans are made to solve them on a priority bases. Those that are critical, which involves safety and welfare of the patient take first priority. Other factors use in determining priority will include severity, frequency, benefit, cost, and liability.

The first step is that the nursing unit must determine how much deviation from the standard is acceptable before changes are made.

In the example of developing a written nursing care plan for every patient as a standard, the unit should decide if 45 out of 50 patients admitted have a care plan recorded within 12 hours of admission and the other 5 have recorded care plans within the next 6 hours, is this deviation acceptable? If not, then how should this be corrected?
- Is the unit short-staffed?
- Have there been an unusually large numbers of admissions recently?
- Are a number of new graduates being oriented on the unit?

After collecting all pertinent information about the possible causes, the nurse manager after consultation with staff and/or supervisor should make plans for correcting deficiencies in performance.

- What needs change? Structural element?
- Process element?
- Outcome element?

Monitoring and Feedback

Follow-up on how effective changes have been in improving performance is very necessary step in the QA process.

If in the example prescribed, the nurse manager found that the next 50 patients had care plans recorded within 12 hours, then the performance had improved relative to that standard. If it had not improved, then another approach would need to be taken, or possibly, the criterion should be evaluated for appropriateness for that unit.

QUALITY ASSURANCE METHODS

The purpose of a nursing QA Program is to measure and improve the quality of patient care delivered in the organization. Therefore, a variety of QA methods have been used. These include:

Nursing Audit

It is a method for evaluating quality of nursing care through the appraisal of the nursing process or customers of care as it is reflected in the patient care records. There are two types of audits:
- Concurrent and
- Retrospective audit.

Peer Review

It is a process by which nurses evaluate one another's job performance against accepted standards.

Patient Care Profiles Analysis

The analysis of longitudinal or cross-sectional complications of data about patients with a particular diagnosis or problem.

Quality Circles

A quality circle is a small group of 5 to 15 employees who perform similar work and meet for one hour each week to solve problems related to their work.

Patient Satisfaction (Client feedback)

Patient satisfaction is used as one of several indicators of quality.

GIVING FEEDBACK TO STAFF

To assure high quality nursing care, information about nursing structure, nursing process and patient outcomes must be continuously feedback to nurses at all levels of organizational hierarchy. Otherwise, faulty practices will persist. Also, reports of favorable findings would be helpful in reinforcing desirable performance by caregivers.

Solve work related problems.

Exercise

Purpose: This session will enable the students.
Analyze communication and group dynamics and conflict resolution patterns.

Directions: The students are assigned to:
- Bring samples of documentation to the class.
- Observe different characteristics of nurses' communication and group dynamics, assertiveness level, professional language used, and general communication skills; of both physicians and nurses.
- Identify common roles played in the group, the missing roles and any impact occur as a result missing communication.
- Identify the sources of conflict and approaches to conflict resolution.
- Get in to groups of 5-8.
- Analyze an example of documentation based on the criteria for proper documentation.
- Ideas to improve communication in your unit based on your observation and class notes.
- To analyze conflict resolution and suggest alternative approaches.
- Develop one scenario on conflict resolution.
- Role play the scenario you developed in front of the class.

Note to the Faculty

- Reinforce the criteria for proper documentation.
- Help in developing the scenarios.
- Give feedback about the role play.

23 Ethics in Managing Health Care

OBJECTIVES
- Define ethics.
- Identify managers obligations related to ethics in health care.
- Identify principles of biomedical ethics.
- Describe the process of dealing with ethical dilemma.

DEFINITION

Ethics is a moral philosophy, a science of judging the relationship of means to ends, and the art of controlling means so they serve human ends. It involves conflict, choice and conscience. The choice is influenced by values, and ethical choices must consider those values together with wants, needs, and rights. A moral dilemma occurs when a decision has equally unsatisfactory alternatives. To make an ethical decision, one must first consider what is found in the means and an end and then determine what good or evil is found in the means and the end.

If a major evil is intended either as means or an end, it is an unethical decision.

ETHICS IN MANAGING HEALTH CARE

Ethics is integral to nursing management and how we operate in a management role is influenced by our values, beliefs, and the experiences that form us as individuals and leaders. Our personal values and the values of the profession in which we have been socialized define responsibilities to our clients and to society. There are different codes and bill of right that could provide framework for making ethical decisions as ANA code for nurses and the social policy statement. The patient bill of rights clarifies rights for patients and implies an obligation on the part of the nurse to assist the patient in securing them.

Manager's Obligation

As one reviews these documents, it is clear that the nurse manager has an obligation to:
- Provide safe and respectful care
- Not discriminate
- Assure privacy and confidentiality
- Ensure that the patient had enough information for informed consent
- Support continuity of care

- Safeguard the public from unethical or illegal practice
- Support the welfare of the profession
- Follow the physician's orders
- Support the policies and procedures of the hospital
- Maintain conditions conducive to high quality
- Collaborate with other health professionals
- Act in accord with one's own values
- Promote the efforts to meet the health needs of the public.

Principles of Biomedical Ethics

Principles of biomedical ethics provide concepts and language that can be used to identify issues, to reflect on them, and to articulate the ethical position we take.

The principle of Autonomy: defined as self-rule or self-governance. Personal autonomy is being one's own person, without constraint, this principle requires that we respect individual in our care as autonomous agent who have the right to control his own life.

The principle of Nonmalefficiency: The principle that requires that we do no harm.
The principle of Beneficience: The doing of good
The principle of Justice: giving each his or her rights and require action that contribute to the welfare of others, and prevention and removal of harm.

A model for addressing ethical issue:
M = massage the dilemma
O = outline options
R = review criteria and resolve
A = affirm position and act
L = look back

Massage the dilemma: To be aware that an ethical dilemma exists. Identify the dilemma and who is, or who should be involved in the process of decision making. Collecting all relevant data possible is the most crucial component of ethical decision making. Identify conflicting wishes and values of each party involved.

Outline options: Clarify options available and the consequences.

Review criteria and resolve: To determine appropriate actions, one must weigh the options against the principles and primary values of those involved. Value consideration for the nurse manager may include: respects staff, acts fairly, etc. Practical consideration such as legal impact, effectiveness and likelihood of success can also be considered. Affirm position and act: decide the next appropriate action and develop a strategy.

Look back: Evaluation of the process, if successful in that it prevented the harm for example or the need to go through the process again.

24 Documentation—Records and Reports

OBJECTIVES
- Describe the types of records and reports available in the nursing unit and their purposes.
- Explain the concept, purposes and kinds of reports.
- Discuss the characteristics of good records and reports.

INTRODUCTION
Records are an account of what has been assessed or observed about a patient and what care has been implemented. They help each health team member to become aware of other member's actions and decisions in delivering care.

DEFINITION
Records are formal legal, administrative tools that permanently document information relevant to direct or indirect patient care.

PURPOSES OF RECORDS
- To communicate with the health team members.
- To educate nursing and medical students.
- To assess patient's condition.
- To protect the hospital from law suits.
- To evaluate quality patient care.
- To be used as a reference for research.

KINDS OF RECORDS
Nursing unit records, i.e. patient's clinical record, nurse's notes, etc.

Nursing office records, i.e. master record of nursing hours, employment records, attendance and personnel records, etc. The discussion in this chapter is mainly on nursing unit records.

NURSING UNIT RECORDS

Types

Patient's Health Care Record or Patient's Chart

It is the most important hospital records. It should be kept with a complete identifying data in a place not available to patients and visitors and protected from loss. Hospitals are legally and ethically obligated to protect the information in patient's records and social workers.

Definition

It is a written record of the diagnostic procedures, the treatment and the progress during hospitalization and patient's condition upon discharge.

Purposes of the Patient's Chart

- It gives an accurate information of the patient's condition and care.
- It aids in diagnosis and treatment of the patient.
- It provides evidence that physician's orders have been carried out and it shows what care has been given, e.g. order for urine analysis after meals, order for suctioning, etc.
- It shows patient's response to his treatment.
- It aids in the detection of changes in patient education, e.g. Laboratory, Investigation Reports and Vital Signs Report, etc.
- It helps in follow up-care.
- It serves as a legal document (Protection for the hospital, physicians and nurses).
- It may be referred to (as a permanent record) in case of subsequent illness.
- It aids in research.

Contents of the Patient's Chart

- Admission and Discharge Record.
- Clinical Examination Record (History and Physical Examination and Continuation Sheet).
- Physician's Order Sheet (Inpatient Drug Prescription Sheet and Intravenous Infusion Therapy).
- Mount Sheet (Laboratory Investigation Report Sheet).
- Nursing Information Sheet and Nursing Care Plan.
- Nursing Progress Sheet or Record (Nurse's Notes).
- Graphic Chart.
- Fluid Balance Chart.

Other Records if Required are

- Diabetic Chart.
- Special Observation Chart.
- Operation/ Procedure Consent Chart, Preoperative Nursing Checklist, Anesthesia Record, Operation Notes.
- *NB:* The contents of the patient's chart are also par of the records available in the nursing unit.

Nursing Progress Sheet or Record (Nurse's Notes)

It is an informative and descriptive record of the nursing care given and includes information and observations of significance so that they can contribute to the continuity of patient care.

It is the only 24 hour nursing record about the patient. Erasing invalidates the record for legal purposes and not acceptable. Errors are indicated by drawing a single line through the word and the nurse signs over it and writes the correction.

Purposes

- Legal proof of what the patient is doing and feeling in the hospital. The physical and mental progress from day-to-day.
- A legal proof of what was performed to the patient during hospitalization on each shift.
- It serves as evidence of either good or negligent practice on the part of the nurse.

Contents

- Identification data (addressograph label).
- Date and time
- Progress report
- Signature

Information given under progress record includes patient's general condition, and any change, special procedures/ treatment performed and its results. Emotional condition, diet, activity, rest and sleep, personal hygiene, elimination, fluid therapy, interaction of family with patients, any nursing measures taken by the nurse during each shift, physician's visit, patient education carried out and any other information significant to patient's condition. Information should be signed after each recording.

NURSING INFORMATION SHEET OR RECORDS

Purpose

To obtain complete data about the patient on admission.

Contents

Admission, Past medical history, Allergies, Admission vital signs, Name band fixed, Physician informed, Valuables, Social assessment, Personal information, Next of kin/ person to contact. Other information and remarks. It should be signed and dated by the admitting nurse.

NURSING CARE PLAN

Purposes

- It provides a guide lines for patient centered care.
- It acts as a means of communication among nursing staff.

- It ensures continuity and quality patient care.
- It acts as a means for evaluating staff performance.

Contents of Nursing Care Plan

- Identification data
- Nursing diagnosis
- Goals
- Nursing orders
- Outcome criteria (Evaluation criteria)

Fluid Balance Chart:

- To assess the fluid and electrolyte balance.
- To aid the physician to identify the imbalance and to prescribe new treatment regimen.
- To assess the patients' condition.

Contents

- Identification data.
- Date and time
- Name of fluid
- Route of intake (oral, I/V, etc.)
- Means of output (Urine, Vomitus, Aspiration, etc.)

Census Record

The nurse in-charge is responsible for making the daily census record on each nursing unit, from which the official census of the hospital is derived. The record shows the number of beds in the unit, the census of patients, and to be revised upon admission, transfer or discharge of a patient. It is sent to the proper administrative office.

Inventory

An itemized record of all furniture, medical and surgical equipment, utensils, instruments, dishes, office and housekeeping equipment, etc. with the necessary identifying data, and the quantity of each article allotted to the unit. Columns are provided for recording the date and the quantity of each article in the unit when an inventory count is taken. An inventory count is taken. An inventory count is made daily, monthly, or periodically according to the items, e.g. thermometers and instrument are counted daily.

Narcotic Record

The first-line nurse manager is responsible for keeping an accurate record of all narcotics received in the nursing unit. A narcotic count should be made at least twice daily.

Other Records

Other records/ forms/ sheets available in the nursing unit and used for the purpose of referral, diet, release of responsibility Against Medical Advice (AMA), Malaria Case Notification, Communicable Diseases-Case Notification, National Program for Prevention and Control of Road Traffic Accidents (RTAs), Accident/ Injury and Death.

REPORTS

Introduction

A full report is given in the morning before distribution of assignment and another time at the end of the shift of duty to the oncoming staff. It includes information about each patient's condition including problems and suggested methods of assisting him/ her as well as his/her treatment and day-to-day progress. Most reports are done orally between the staff and certain reports need to be written.

Definition

A report is a system of communication aimed at transferring essential information necessary for safe and holistic patient care.

Purposes

- To communicate progress of the patient's health status to all nurses in different shift.
- To prepare staff members for their day's work.
- To ensure that all members of the health care team have the same information.
- To provide quality and continuity of care from one shift to the next.

KINDS OF REPORTS

Oral

They are given when the information is for immediate use and not for permanency. They may be based on material included in a written report.
- Reports between the head nurse (nurse in-charge) and her assistant, e.g. patients' conditions, treatment, medications, observations, admissions, discharges.
- Reports between nurses who are assigned to bedside care.
- Reports of staff members to the charge nurse: During the day and when on duty, e.g. patients' conditions, results of treatment carried out, etc.
- Nurse in-charge reports to bedside nurses, e.g. change in orders.
- Report of the charge nurse to the nurse supervisor: It includes names, diagnosis, treatment of each patient, condition, problem in nursing care, complaints, general picture of the unit.
- Reports of the charge nurse to the clinical instructor, e.g. similar to supervisor in addition to student progress.

- Report of the Supervisor to the Director of Nursing (Nursing Officer): Similar to the supervisor.
- Report of the charge nurse to the physician, e.g. patient's symptoms, results of treatment, complaints, problems, etc.
- A report can be given orally in person or by audiotape. An in-person report permits nurse to obtain immediate feedback about unclear or incomplete information. The report may be conducted in the conference room or during nurse's "walking rounds".

Written Reports

Census Report

Daily census or the number of patients in the nursing unit at midnight.

Reports on Mistakes and Accidents

Accurate and comprehensive reports on both the patients charts and in the accident report is essential to protect the hospital (documentation for legal consequences), For examples: medication errors, falls, refusal of treatment, or to sign consent for treatment, complications from procedures, dissatisfaction with care, etc. What happens to the patient may be an accident but the telling or reporting of this is an incident. It is also called as incidental or anecdotal report and helps for staff appraisal.

Change of Shift Reports: (The unit report or hand over)
(Day, evening and night reports)

The change of shift report or inter-shift report occurs three times a day in every type of nursing unit in all types of health care settings. At the end of shift, nurses share information about their assigned clients to the nurses working on the next shift.

Purpose: To provide continuity of care from one shift to the next.
Examples of information to be included in the report:
- Day, date, time, shift.
- Patient's name, age, diagnosis.
- Nursing problems.
- Description of patient's physiological and psychological conditions.
- Tests, procedures, or surgery scheduled.
- New therapies ordered.
- Dietary restrictions, teaching plan.
- Patient's response to nursing care measures.
- Admissions, discharges, seriously ill patients and transfers from and to the unit.

Inter-departmental Reports

For example: Reports to the admitting office and information desk of patients to be discharged, medicolegal cases, clients needing social support and extended health services.

Patient's safety: The nurse follows the agency's policy about the frequency of documenting and adjust the frequency as patient's condition indicates.

Documenting should also be done as soon as possible after an assessment or intervention by the person assessing.

Confidentiality

The patient's record is protected legally as a private record of the patient's care. Access to the record is only allowed to health professionals involved in giving care to the patient and not to significant others or any person. A patient who is making a claim for compensation may ask to have the medial history used as evidence. In this instance, the patient must sign an authorization for review, copying, or release of information from the record. This form clearly indicates what information is to be released to whom.

For purposes of education and research, most agencies allow students and graduate health professionals access to patients records. The records are used in patient conferences, clinics, rounds and written papers or patient studies. The student or graduate is bound by a strict ethical code to hold all information in confidence.

Permanence

All entries on the patient's record are made in dark-colored ink so that the record is permanent and changes can be identified. Dark-colored ink is generally required because it reproduces well on microfilm and in duplication processes. Entries need to be legible hand printing or easily understood handwriting is usually permissible. Nurses should follow the agency's policies about the type of pen used for documenting.

Accuracy

It is essential that notations on records be accurate and correct. Accurate notations consist of facts or exact observations, rather than opinions or interpretations of an observations, which will be more accurate.

For Example

A nurse records on kardex to that *the patient "was uncooperative"* to carry out a procedure, which is her opinions or an interpretations which may or may not be accurate.

Similarly, when a patient expresses his worry about the diagnosis or problem. This should be quoted directly on the record as Mr. S *"stated that he is worried about his leg"*.

Principles to be kept in mind while documenting the patient condition:

- Nurses should record exactly whatever they hear as well as what they observe.
- When describing something, nurses should also avoid general words, such as large, good, or normal, which can be interpreted differently by different persons.
- Correct spelling is essential for accuracy in documenting. When the nurse makes a recording error in charting, the nurse draws a line through it and writes the word error above it, with the nurse's initials or name depending on agency policy.

- Errors should not be erased.
- If a blank space is left after completion of documentation the nurse needs to draw a line through the blank space so that no additional information can be recorded at any other time or by any other person, and signs the notation at end.
- In any case the policy of the agency needs to be checked.
- Correction fluid should not be used to erase anything documented.

Example 1

Doctors prescription says that " Dress the wound with saline - OD"

If a nurse writes on the nurses progress record/kardex as dressing is done with betadine when the prescription is with the saline in order to do the correction. Just she needs to cross the line through the word as shown (Sally) then write as saline and place signature clearly.

Example 2

Ordering diet for the patients in the ward:

After completing the diet sheet for few patients requiring diet from the hospital if there is an empty space in the sheet, draw a line across to prevent any entries later on and avoid errors.

MODEL OF PREPARING A DIET SHEET

Bed. No. 21.   Time: 10 AM   Ward: Female medical

Sl. No	Name of the patient	Hospital no:	Diagnosis	Diet requested
1.	Mrs. Sally George	NJ007	DM	1500cal
2.	Mrs. Karen	NJ017	Hypertension	Salt free diet

Signature of the Staff Nurse: Ms.M

Date: 21.6.07

Example 3

Sample recoding of patient teaching:
- Date: 8.5.96/Time: 11 am
- Mr. S is taught on the need for personal cleanliness to prevent wound infection.
- Sign: Ms. S. Carol (RN)

Sequence

The nurse documents events in the order in which they occur. For example, the nurse records assessments, then the nursing interventions, and then the patient's responses.

Appropriateness

Only information that pertains to the patient's health problems and care is recorded. Any other personal information that the patient conveys to the nurse is inappropriate unless it had a direct bearing on the patient's health problem.

Completeness

Not all data that a nurse obtains about a patient can be recorded. Also, the information that is recorded needs to be complete and helpful to the patient and health care professionals. For example, the nurse describes nursing care administered and the patients' response.

The Use of Standard Terminology

The nurse needs to use only commonly accepted abbreviations, symbols, and terms that are specified by the agency or internationally accepted.

Example 4

Mrs. Y is posted for surgery C/M (coming morning) instead of stating as tomorrow at 10 am.

C/M is not used as commonly accepted abbreviations, should avoid such confusing documentation, hospital policies need be followed.

Brevity

Recordings need to be brief as well as complete, to save time in communication. The patient's name and the word patient are omitted. For example, the nurse may write "Perspiring profusely, Respiration's shallow, 28/min". Each thought or sentence is terminated with a period.

Each recording on the nursing notes is signed by the nurse making it. The signature includes the name and title, for example, "Mary Ann Thomas, RN" Nurses need to follow agency policy about how to sing their names. Some agencies permit initials rather than first name (e.g. MA Thomas). The following title abbreviations are often used, but nurses are advised to check the practice in their agencies.

RN   -   Registered nurse
RM   -   Registered Midwife
St/N -   Student Nurse

25. Change Process—Planned Change

OBJECTIVES

- Explain the concept of planned change.
- Discuss reasons and phases of change, driving and restraining forces and strategies for planned change.
- Describe the process of planned change.
- Identify the skill of the change agent.

INTRODUCTION

Change is inevitable in any organization with advancement of science and technology and revolution in information systems, a nurse manager is constantly confronted with new challenges. Change should not be viewed as a threat but as a challenge or chance to do something new and innovative. Change should only be implemented for good reasons.

DEFINITION

Planned change is a change that results from a well thought out and deliberate effort to make something happen. It is the deliberate application of knowledge and skills by a leader to bring about a change (Tappen 1995).

A change agent is the person responsible for moving others – who are affected by the change – through the stages of change.

STAGES OF PLANNED CHANGE

Lewin (1951), identified three phases through which the change agent must proceed before a planned change becomes part of the system. These stages are:

Unfreezing

In this phase, the change agent unfreezes the forces that maintain status quo. It is the responsibility of the change agent – after thorough and accurate assessment – to convince the people for the need to change. It is also possible that the people themselves are discontented and aware of a need to change.

Moving

In this phase the change agent identifies plans and implements appropriate change strategies ensuring that the driving forces exceed restraining forces. Whenever possible the change should be implemented gradually.

Refreezing

In this phase, the change agent assists in stabilizing the system change so that it becomes integrated and remains so.

The driving and restraining forces for change (Marriner-Tomey 1992).

Driving forces	Restraining forces
Pressure from manager	Continuity to norms, morals and ethics
Desire to please manager	Desire for security
Perception that change will improve self image	Perception of threat-economic or prestige and homeostasis
Belief that change will improve situation	Regulatory mechanisms for keeping the situation fairly constant.

According to Sullivan and Decker 1988, the reasons for effecting change are:
1. To solve a problem.
2. To increase efficiency and effectiveness.
3. To reduce unnecessary workload.

There are three different types of change strategies which can be used to effect change (Bennis, Benne and Chinn 1969).

Rational – empirical strategy: This strategy is used when there is little or no resistance to change. Change is perceived as reasonable by the effected people, when given factual information documenting the need for change.

Normative – reductive strategy: This strategy is used when there is resistance to change due to uncertainty or lack of knowledge. The group process and peer pressure are used to effect change. Group norms are used to socialize and influence individuals so that change will occur.

Power – coercive strategy: This strategy is used only when the resistance is great and irrational. It requires application of power by legitimate authority in order to effect change.

Planned Change

Identify the Problem or Opportunity

Opportunities demand change as the problems, but most managers overlook these opportunities. Change is often planned to close a performance gap, a discrepancy between the desired and the actual state of affairs.

Whether it's a problem or opportunity, it must be identified clearly by asking the following questions: where we are now? what is unique about us? what can we do that is different and better? what is the deriving forces in our organization? what prevent us from moving? what kind of change is required?.

Collect Data

Once the problem or opportunity is clearly defined, the change agent collects data needed. This step is important to the later success in the planned change.

All deriving and restraining forces are identified so that the deriving forces can be strengthened and restraining forces are identified so that the deriving forces can be strengthened and restraining forces reduced.

It is imperative to assess the political pulse.
- Who will gain from this change?
- Who will lose?
- Which of these has more power and why?
- Can those power bases be altered how?
- Who is in control?

It is also important to assess the commitment of the involved people, the structure and the processes of the organization, cost and benefit analyses and resources.

Analyze Data

Collecting good data is important, but it's as important to analyze the data into useful information to make important decisions.

The point is to flush out the resistance.

Identify potential solutions and strategies.

Begin to identify areas of consensus and build a case for the selected option.

Whenever possible, a need to persuade persons in power who are comfortable with financial analyses, statistics and probabilities.

The idea is to develop and present strong argument to support suggested change.

Plan the Change Strategy

Planning "who, how, and when" of the change is a key step.

What will be the target system for change? Members from this system should be involved in this planning stage, and the more involved they are at this point, the less resistance there will be later.

Present attitudes, habits, and ways of thinking have to soften so members of the target system will be ready for the change and dissatisfaction to the present system should be developed by introducing information.

Anxiety about the change should be minimized. There is a need to plan the resources required and establish feedback mechanisms to evaluate the progress in the change by setting goals with specific time frames and identifying indicators for evaluation.

Implement Change

- The plans are put into motion.
- Interventions are designed to gain necessary compliance.
- The change agent creates supportive climate, acts as energizer, obtain and provide feedback and overcome resistance.

At this point there might be a need for providing information, training, discussions, or counseling to change individuals' perceptions, attitudes, values and develop necessary skills.

Evaluate Effectiveness

The established operational indicators are monitored and the extent of success and failure is determined and explained.

Stabilize the Change

Support System for the Change is Developed

To assure permanency of change, through continuous feedback, reinforcement and providing the necessary policies, procedures, standard, etc.

The Change Agent Skills

Successful change agent demonstrates certain characteristics that can be cultivated and mastered with practice.
Among these characteristics are:
- The ability to combine ideas,
- The ability to energize others,
- Skills in human relations,
- Integrative thinking,
- Flexibility to modify ideas,
- Persistent, confidence, realistic thinking,
- Trustworthy,
- Ability to articulate a vision, and
- Ability to handle resistance.

Class room Exercise 1: Analysis of the First-line Nurse Manager's Role

Guidelines for Assignment.

Objective

Imagine that you were asked to study the unit you are working in to identify methods to produce better patient out comes, to do that you need to analyze your work setting with in the system framework.
Consider the following guidelines in analyzing your work setting and write your recommendations:
- *Identify:* Philosophy, objectives, standards, organizational structure, communication lines, management style.
- Analyze the relationship between the nursing department and nursing unit in relation to what you identified above.
- Identify the main processes carried out in your work setting.

- Discuss the quality assurance process at the nursing department level and at the unit level.
- Indicate the important outcome indicators for your work setting.
- Write your recommendations to improve patient outcomes based on the analyses you made.

Your assignment should be typed (single spaced), not less than three pages.
Documents supporting your argument should be included in the appendices.
The overall presentation of the paper is important.
Evaluation will be based on the following criteria: depth, comprehensiveness and presentation.

Exercise 2: Introducing Change

Guideline for Assignment

Choose any area you think that your nursing unit needs to change to improve the unit, and to produce better patient outcomes.

Write Clearly your Suggested Change

Imagine that you want to submit a proposal with this suggested change to the higher management, develop a convincing proposal considering the change theory, and supporting your argument with: statistics, incident reports, feedback from nurses and management, evaluation or quality assurance reports, research studies and any reference you find useful. Include the following in your proposal.

Analyses of the current situation, the problem area that requires the suggested change and the situation surrounding it.

Explain clearly how you are going to introduce this change, develop a plan, provide a summarized action plan at the end of this part including: objectives, strategies, time period and distribution of responsibilities.

Explain how you are going to follow-up on your change, develop evaluation and follow-up plan.

Develop your cost estimate for this change project, you can work with the in-charge to do that or ask a financial person.

Part C: Management of Nursing Educational Institutions

Unit IX: Program Planning

26 Development of Program Objective

INTRODUCTION

An institute is described as an organization that has particular purpose especially one that is connected with education or a particular profession. An institution is referred to a large important organization that has particular purpose, e.g. university where education is offered. Nursing institutes are those which offer nursing education of various programs. Such as general nursing program, Baccalaureate program, master degree in nursing or doctoral degree in nursing.

The tasks involved in planning and conducting an educational program can be classified into four major types, namely:

- Deciding on the objectives.
- Selecting learning experiences that will contribute to the objectives.
- Organizing the learning experiences to maximize their cumulative effect.
- Evaluating the effectiveness of the educational program in attaining its objectives through appraising the educational progress of the students.

Education is a process for changing the behavior of students in desired directions. The term "behavior" is used in the broad sense and includes thinking, feeling and acting.

It is clear that the educational objectives are the behavior patterns that the school tries to develop in the student. The only rational basis for selecting learning experiences and devising evaluation procedures is in terms of their relation to the educational objectives.

The second major task of education is to select learning experiences that will contribute to the objectives. "People acquire them by practicing them".

A student develops understanding by recalling ideas, by explaining them in his own words, and by finding illustrations of them. Skill in ways of thinking is developed by practicing problem-solving again and again. An attitude is acquired as the student looks repeatedly at the phenomenon from a new perspective. Interests are required by getting satisfaction from certain kinds of experiences so that the experiences become increasingly satisfying. For all of these kinds of behavior, students acquire new behavior patterns by practicing them.

One fact clearly emerges from this analysis—the teacher cannot learn for the student. To plan learning experiences is to outline the activities that will give the students a chance to practice the behavior implied by the objectives. Thus, planning a particular course will mean providing situations in which the students will encounter problems to solve so that they can gain understanding and develop critical thinking.

The third major task in education is to organize the learning experiences to maximize their cumulative effect.

The fourth major task in education is to evaluate the effectiveness of the educational program in attaining its objectives, through appraising the educational progress of the students. It means appraisal early in the course as well as near the end. It involves evidence relating to all of the important objectives which will help us to identify those aspects of the curriculum that are effective and those that need improving.

OBJECTIVES OF PROFESSIONAL EDUCATION

The development of an ethical practitioner who has an adequate understanding of the ethical code of the profession, who applies the ethical principles intelligently to the varied particular instances that arise, and who is sincerely committed to the highest ends of the profession, requires an education program which consciously aims at several major types of objectives.

In terms of knowledge and understanding, a program of professional education needs to develop in students a broad and clear concept of the social role of their profession.

Also, in terms of knowledge and understanding, professional education aims at developing a deep understanding of the persons to whom the professional service is rendered, including particularly insight into personal motivations, feelings, needs, and the inter-relation of physical, psychological, social, and emotional aspects of human behavior.

In terms of effective thinking or problem solving, the objectives of professional education which are derived from the importance of ethics include the ability to recognize ethical problems, the ability to identify the ethical principles at issues, and the ability to work out appropriate courses of action in terms of ethical principles.

In terms of attitudes, education for the profession aims at developing loyalty to the social well-being of the persons who are served by the profession, concern for a truly social role on the part of the profession, a sense of self-respect for the social contributions of his profession and of his own work, and a warm, accepting, yet objective attitude towards his clients. This involves developing in professional students a considerable degree of emotional maturity so that they are free to express and receive emotionally charged communication and at the same time can act intelligently as new problem arise.

Finally, of course, every professional school needs to aim consciously to develop any understanding of those principles, concepts, facts, and procedures which are basic to professional operations. In medicine these include principles of physiology, anatomy, chemistry, physics, bacteriology, and psychology. The tendency, however, is to limit these basic principles too narrowly. In a very real sense, doctors deal with problems in their normal professional work which are psychological and require an understanding of relevant psychological principles if they are to operate intelligently.

In terms of effective thinking and problem-solving, it is clear that foregoing objectives involving knowledge imply the development of some skill in recognizing professional problems, in analyzing the problems in terms of the relevant principles, and in working out courses of action by applying these principles.

In terms of attitudes, the use of principles, rather than rules, in a profession requires as objectives in professional education the development of broad, rather than narrow interest in the fields on which the profession draws, and the development of the student's interest in continuing his own learning long after graduation from a professional's school.

PLANNING LEARNING EXPERIENCES

The most common problems in professional schools in connection with the learning experiences used are:
- The failure to select learning experiences in terms of the objectives to be attained.
- The failure to utilize consciously appropriate learning procedures for developing problem-solving skills, attitudes, and interest.
- The failure to develop effective motivation for learning.

These are serious deficiencies.

Since learning is an active process, in which the learner himself is definitively involved, motivation is essential. Since the learner learns more than knowledge of content and he actually learns what he is doing, what he is feeling, what he is thinking, it is important to make conscious plans for students to learn to solve problems, to develop attitudes and interests.

Understanding the social functions the profession serves and how these functions are related to the total functioning of society and to the functions of other major specialized groups. It is to serve as a guide for planning learning, we must have a clear idea of what is meant by "understanding" as a type of behavior to be developed and what content is included in the phrase beginning "the social functions the profession serves". Most instructors who have sought to define "understanding" indicate that it is a mental process that is more active than memorization, since it involves not only remembering but also the ability to explain the concept or principle in one's own words, the ability to interpret, to illustrate, and to compare and contrast it to related ideas.

Correspondingly, as we define each objective in terms of the behavior and content implied, it is a much easier step to select learning experiences that give students a chance to practice the behavior involved and to utilize the relevant content. In this way, learning experiences are planned in terms of the objectives sought. Interests in certain kinds of activities are developed as the student gains satisfaction from participating in these activities. Since the learner learns through his reactions, unless he can be guided to be think, feel, and act in ways appropriate to the situation, it is not possible to learn for him. Practice alone, even when carried out to unusual limits, does not take the place of the learners being involved in what he is doing.

ORGANIZING LEARNING EXPERIENCE

It is necessary that what is learned this term builds upon what was learned last term, that what will be learned next year builds upon what is learned this year. This is sequence of learning.

It includes variety in the learning experiences, so that each subsequent term emphasizes the main things to be learned, but in varied contexts. In this way, ever broader and deeper learning are achieved.

Furthermore, effective organization provides for relating one course to another and one field to another, which reinforces the learning in each course or field in another. This is done both by helping the student to use things learned in one course or field in another, and by helping him to perceive differences as well as similarities in the concepts, principles, attitudes and skills utilized in various courses and fields. This is called curriculum integration.

Sequence and integration are essential to programs of professional education, but because of the tendency towards specialization and separation, conscious efforts are required to plan for and develop effective organization.

Another effort at extending the sequential organization of professional education is the working out of definite plans for continuing education after the members of the profession has completed pre-service training and has been inducted into the initial activities of his work.

Now there is marked tendency for professional schools to develop programs of continuing education, in some cases brining the work of the school to the practitioner in the field, in other cases setting up short courses, institutes, or long-term seminars for practitioners to take on the campus.

EVALUATING EFFECTIVENESS OF EDUCATIONAL PROGRAMS

The final attributes of professional education are those involved in the task of evaluating the effectiveness of the educational programme in attaining its objectives, through appraising the educational progress of the students.

Important attributes are too often neglected in current educational programs.

The **first** of these is conducting an appraisal in terms of all of the important educational objectives of the professional schools.

The **second** attribute, often neglected, may partly account for the shortcomings in the first. A comprehensive program of evaluation uses varied devices for obtaining evidence regarding the educational progress of students. These device include not only written tests and examinations, useful as they are, but also observations, interviews, questionnaires, reports from the field and samples of the students work; in short, any device which gives valid evidence regarding the significant behavior of the students. This does not provide adequate means for comprehensive evaluation.

The four 'C's of curriculum planning:
1. **Cooperative:** A program prepared jointly by a group of persons will be less liable to error than one prepared by a single person.

2. **Continuous:** The preparation of a program is not a one-shot operation. In planning it, provision should be made for its continuing revision.
3. **Comprehensive:** In an approach which accepts the interaction of all the program components, each must be defined with the requisite precision.
4. **Concrete:** General and abstract considerations are not a sufficient basis for drawing up a program. Concrete professional tasks must constitute the essential structure of a relevant program.

—Adapted from E. Krug

The vision of Ralph W. Tyler is valid till today as **For those concerned in curriculum planning clearly means that the order of the day is patience and perseverance.**

So, a program describes as a series of planned educational activities a student need to go through with the assistance of teachers. In order to ensure the harmonious functioning of the educational process for more effective training, **Integration of a curriculum** coordination of different teaching/learning activities is important.

27 Trends and Issues in Nursing Curriculum Development

INTRODUCTION

If one is to be a educator, one must be a learner, and if one is to educate in a democracy. One must live by its principles. Education is not just a job- it is a way of life.

J LANIER AND P CUSIK (1986)

So, the object of education is not to "shape citizens to the uses of society, but to produce citizens to shape a better society". Every individual should have access to a type of education that permits maximum development of his potential and capabilities. Thus, education is a process, the chief goal of which is to bring about change in the behavior of the student in the course of a given period of time.

So, the important process of educating graduate nursing students is development of curriculum there can be no question of continuing to copy the models of the past, or in the case of developing countries, foreign models. The educational system leading to the development of health personnel at all levels must be re-examined with in the context of the needs of the country concerned (WHO offset publication no: 35).

In order to develop the nursing curriculum the following trends and issues need to be understood by the educators of nursing.

DEFINITION OF TERMS

1. **Trend:** Trend is an event that occurs over that occurs overtime and shows a series of fluctuation in its patterns.
   (Stanhope Lancaster)
   Trend is a change which takes place consciously in an informal way over the years.
   (Collins GEM dictionary)
2. **Issue:** An issue is a topic of interest which leads into a discussion and requiring a decision.
3. **Curriculum:** Curriculum is a specified course of study.
   (Collins GEM dictionary)
   Curriculum is referred to the subjects that are included in a course of study or taught in a school, college, etc.
   (Oxford dictionary)
   Now let us focus on the following important T R E N D S

CLASSIFICATION OF TRENDS

1. Societal trends
2. Science and technological trends

3. General educational trends
4. Trends in the health care systems
5. Trends in the nursing education and nursing practice.

Social Trends

Deals with growing needs and existing health situation of the country. The most important quality in an educational program is its relevance. Training program for health personnel must enable the graduates to cope effectively with the problems they will encounter in the context of their work.

a. Therefore, the first step is to identify and analyze the health problems of the community so as to enable to define the communities health needs, priorities and casual analysis. These elements will serve as the starting point for the design of an educational program.
b. The country has to develop policy orientation to health problems in accordance with the international standards and standards set by WHO.
c. Review existing national plans in relation to health, nutrition, agriculture or education in order to derive an idea of the country's general goals for health.

So, assessing the health situation of the country is an important and first element in curriculum development.

Science and Technological Trends

The second element which draws the attention of educators is the advancement in science and technology in the global context and the position of the country.

Any program of action intended to improve the health situation in a society at the national, district, local, family or individual level must be able to draw support from different sectors. Specially regarding invention of high tech equipment, i.e. biomedical technology in the provision of secondary and tertiary care for clients. Both in the hospital and for home care management.

For example, all the equipment are computerized such as monitors, therapy appliances, scanners for diagnostic purposes and computers for storage of information. So it is an essential aspect to be kept in mind in the development of curriculum in order to prepare competent nurses.

General Educational Trends

Educational institutions are one of the support systems for health care activities. This system is responsible for education and training from the primary level to the university level and beyond. It is important that it should function well, as it must supply human resources with the skills needed by the other support system. So it is important that the existence of an efficient educational system in a prerequisites for any action to improve the health situation in a country.

For example, twelve years of schooling with preparation of basic general sciences as prerequisites to enter any professional courses and school education should enable the students to go up in the ladder of higher education.

Trends in the Health Care System

In the present world health care system has become more complex entity with its growing subsystem and super specialty in all the branches of medical care. So it is essential to understand the actors involved in and the activities related to health care, i.e. the participants involved in activities related to health care both in the health system and support system.

There are two types of actors. providers of health care and users of health services. They will produce valuable feedback for those whose task is to design training program for health personnel. Direct providers of health care are doctors and nurses. Indirect providers of health care are inter professional groups including other health personnel.

For example, community medicine, family medicine, genetics and counseling community health nursing, geriatric nursing and occupational nursing, etc. as growing specialties in the health care system and in nursing.

Trends in Nursing Education and Nursing Practice

a. *Nursing Education:* The form of teaching has remained unchanged for centuries. The needs of society. The practical side of the matter have been left to chance, whereas specific features of the situation of each country are changing more rapidly. Unfortunately, little or no account has been taken in to consideration for the training of health personnel, but following traditional systems in teaching. What is required now is to make sure that the educational program are relevant?
No educational system can be effective unless its purposes are clearly defined.

The members of health team must be trained specially for the task they will have to perform taking into account the circumstances under which they will work, so defining the professional task of health personnel to be trained is the very basis of the educational objectives of training centers/institutions and must be shaped selectively in terms of the goal to be achieved. If the goal is modified in the course of time the program also to be modified accordingly.

Definition of professional task must proceed from a study of needs, availability of resources, various category of personnel be called upon to do their professional career in a given type of health services. In nursing education, depending upon the needs of the country we need to deicide whom we would like to prepare, the type of health services to be provided and to achieve the institutional goal and educational objectives.

For example, generalist or specialist such as graduate midwives, lactation consultants, birth spacing consultants, etc. Depending on these professional task to be identified and prepare the suitable educational objectives and educational programmers as pre-registration nursing courses for diploma level and post-registration courses for the higher education framework with the pathways leading towards an honors degree or masters and doctoral degree.

b. *Nursing Practice:* Definition of professional task become precondition for ensuring that the training program are really designed to meet the population health needs. The training programs, professional profile and educational program objectives should provide basis for nursing practice in all three levels of health care. such as primary, secondary and tertiary health care. The advancement to adopted and develop professional skill as specialist is essential. So that the nurses can be prepared as clinical consultants, administrators and as researches in the various fields of nursing practice in order to make both nursing education and practice identical three principles are fundamental importance.

It must be oriented towards the community as well as the individuals taking account of the needs of each particular activity, i.e. education must be community oriented.

The education must be learner centered. If educational objectives are based on faulty principles, then the "best system" of training may give "bad results".

The support system which should support health systems are:
- The political system
- The structure and authorities of the administrative system
- The general system/general infrastructure
- The education system

Unfortunately, most of the time these systems act as obstacles rather than support.

Based upon these trends the following issues need to be looked into before developing curriculum.

ISSUES

1. Where are we now?

As nursing faculty we need to answer the question and analyze the present situation whether or not we are on the road to relevant, which means the validation of curriculum or judgmental process in which an attempt is to be made to ascribe a degree of worth or value to a curriculum (wells 1987) in the context of professional education and preparation of participants for their professional role.

Walker describes five types of validation.
a. Academic validation
b. Professional validation
c. Economic validation
d. Institutional validation
e. Performance validation

Then identify the strengths of present system/situation before starting the program.

2. Where we want to go?

This deals with the thinking and aspiration for future. Faculty must think whether the educational program what is designed will help to meet the expectations of individuals, families and communities in accordance far with the developed countries or not.

3. What we want to achieve?

Nurse educators must be able to analyze and think critically that we are preparing the students with the adequate skills to perform their expected roles in all the three domains of professional tasks such as practical, communication and intellectual skills according to the institutional goals and educational objectives.

The three types of skills to be achieved.
- Domain of attitudes (communication skills)
  For example, Feelings, values and interpersonal relationships
- Domain of practical skills (imitation control and automatism)
- Domain of intellectual skills (knowledge and recall of facts)
  For example, Interpretation of data and problem solving.

4. How can we achieve?

The faculty must think the ways by which the curriculum can be developed to which is relevant to meet the needs of the country.

Dr. Alan Myles describes curriculum can be developed in four phases:

1. *Initiation phase:*
   - During this phase curriculum development groups or course planning teams need to identify the priorities for course development.
   - General nursing course or specialty nursing course.
   - Increased competitiveness.
   - Different education institutions biding for student numbers.
   - Ex: the number of intake of students for each course need to identify whether they are demand—led or resource led.
     Whether it is safer to start the program.

2. *Development phase:* During this phase new modules and courses are developed. Important decisions made during this phase concerned with:
   - Precise educational objectives of the course.
   - Selection/rejection of the content for the scheme of study.
   - Modes of teaching and learning.
   - Scheme of assessment.
     In this phase it may be false perception than a reality. May be ideal but not practical.

3. *Implementation phase:* This refers to the curriculum and associated materials in action. Still it may differ significantly from the formal curriculum the actual experience of students and teachers may be quite different from that described in the definitive course document.

4. *Evaluation phase:* (it should be on going)
   - General aspects of an education provider and proposed curriculum
   - Rationale and Philosophy
   - Scheme of study – duration of the study period
   - Modes of teaching and learning
   - Scheme of assessment.

5. *When can we achieve the desired goal?*
   This deals with the time frame of the program to be completed.
   Then assess the program at the end of implementation of curriculum.

After understanding the trends and issues of the health care and health status of the country the faculty must decide to understand the mission, philosophy, and objectives of the program and the educational institution. Then develop educational objectives.

The essentials needed to develop a curriculum include:
- Mission statement of the educational institutions
- Identification of philosophy
- Educational concepts
- Educational models
- Educational theories
- Standards of global education.

Once these are accepted by all educational authorities and the faculty involved, implementation of curriculum is facilitated.

Based on these trends and issues the nursing curriculum to be developed to suit or to meet the needs of individuals, families and country and the international standards of nursing education and practice.

Unit X: Planning and Organization of Curriculum

28 Curriculum Planning

INTRODUCTION

Concepts regarding the meaning of curriculum, its purpose, nature and who should be involved in its development change from time-to-time. The story of curriculum development in education in general and in nursing education in particular might be considered as a history of the evolution and the revolution of the curriculum in achieving and maintaining a balance between the ends and the means of education.

Fox identified four positions regarding the meaning of intellectual development as a purpose of the curriculum. Which have relevance for nursing education.

1. Intellectual development is conceived as a mastery of subject matter achieved primarily through teacher exposition, drills, tests, etc. The traditional subject matter curriculum is an example of this concept. The early nursing curricula were essentially of this type. The so called "formal classes" – doctor's, lectures and nurses' classes constituted the nursing curriculum. And even though students were placed in clinical setting for experience, this was looked upon as clinical practice and in many cases simply as work experience and not as a part of the curriculum.

2. Intellectual development is conceived as a being directed toward the development of the process itself, i.e. problem solving, and creative thinking, etc. mastery of subject matter in and of itself is secondary. However, more emphasis is given frequently to problems than to the process of problem-solving. Hence, the structures of these curricula really have not been altered very much. They remain essentially subject-matter curricula.

3. Intellectual development of an individual is related to and dependent on the development of all aspects of personality. Growth of the learner is inter-related emotional health, personal and social adjustment, skill in group interaction, physical health – all contribute and are essential to intellectual effectiveness. As co-curricular activities, student government, social clubs and dormitory living are required.

    Emphasis on the inclusion of: (1) subject matter and directed learning experiences relating to interpersonal relations, (2) more and better use of group techniques, and (3) widening the nursing students contact with students and teachers outside of the health field area few evidences of consideration of this approach to curriculum development in nursing.

4. Intellectual development is important, but development for effective functioning in all areas of living is important in and of itself; therefore, the school has a responsibility to provide for the students development for citizenship, parenthood,

religious development, etc. The issue with arises here is to what extent the school should assume responsibility for development in these areas, or are also it is the responsibilities of the home, the church, the community.

The essential purpose of a school of basic nursing is to prepare a practitioner of nursing. Therefore, primary emphasis in the curriculum will be on nursing and related field.

The school of nursing preparing the professional practitioner of nursing must be concerned with the development of a nurse who will be interested in the health and the related aspects of the community and will assume responsibility for contributing towards the improvement of health of the community as well as of individual to whom she may give nursing care. This means that the school must provide opportunities for the development of knowledge, skills and attitudes which make this possible. Consequently this approach has relevance for nursing education.

Levels of Curriculum Planning

There are three levels of curriculum planning. (Fig. 28.1) They are:

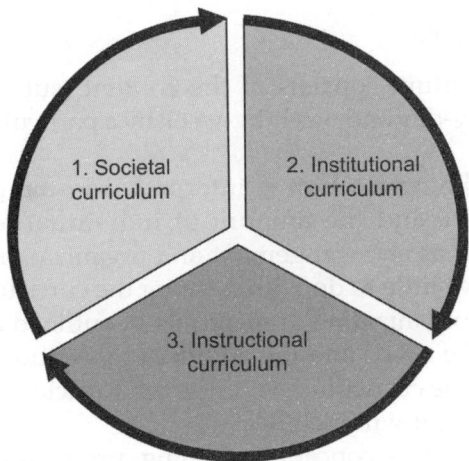

Fig. 28.1: Levels of curriculum planning

Societal Curriculum

A societal curriculum refers to the curricula or parts of curricula which are planned for a large group or class of students. It's the curriculum planned by groups outside of an educational institution. There are many groups exert pressure on curriculum development in schools. First there are the groups set up by national organization such as the council of member agencies of the Department of Baccalaureate and higher degrees, INC, National League for Nursing, who determined criteria which shall be used in the accreditation of educational institutions. These groups are more immediately concerned with determining general characteristics of curriculum content, sequence and implementation, which are likely to prepare the type of nurse practitioner needed to meet society's needs for nursing. Such decisions are so broad and complex that they call for planning on a national level; they couldn't be resolved satisfactorily on an individual basis. Lastly, government at both the national and state levels also can influence curriculum development in educational institutions. The base of curriculum planning and organization in each situation should still be determined by the faculty of each educational institution.

The Institutional Curriculum

The institutional curriculum is one planned by a faculty for a clearly identified group of students, who will spend a specified time period in a particular institution. It is generally referred to when one speaks of a curriculum in a particular school.

The need for and the importance of cooperative planning through curriculum committee within the school is obvious if one looks at the broad base of facts, principles, understandings, skills, habits, attitudes and appreciations that are required to prepare the student to function as a modern professional nurse in a democratic society (To insert example).

The Instructional Curriculum

The instructional curriculum consists of the content (subject matter and learning activities) planned day-by-day and week-by-week by a particular teacher for a particular group of students.

The way in which the curriculum is interpreted in the particular situation will influence the importance and the amount of individual teacher planning. If the curriculum is interpreted as an arrangement and organization of subject matter only, then the teacher may have little to do with forming the curriculum. Under this concept she may use simply the organization of materials as outlined and plan around subject matter independent of the needs and the abilities of the students.

On the other hand, if the curriculum is conceived to include all the planned learning experiences of the student, it will include:
1. Essential facts, information, concepts, meaning, principles.
2. Activities that are necessary for the development of skills, habits, attitudes, ideals, appreciations.
3. Methods that are useful in teaching, supervising, guiding and evaluating results.

Therefore, such concept of curriculum includes all the content planned by the teacher and/or the students and experienced by the students to achieve in the students the desired behavior changes implicit in the educational objectives.

Major Factors which Influence Curriculum Development in Nursing Education

The major factors which influence the curriculum development in the school of nursing are:
1. Philosophy of nursing education
2. Educational psychology

3. Society
4. The student
5. Life activities
6. Knowledge

In addition to the six general factors, one additional factor – that of resources-remains as a primary factor influencing the development of a specific curriculum (Fig. 28.2).

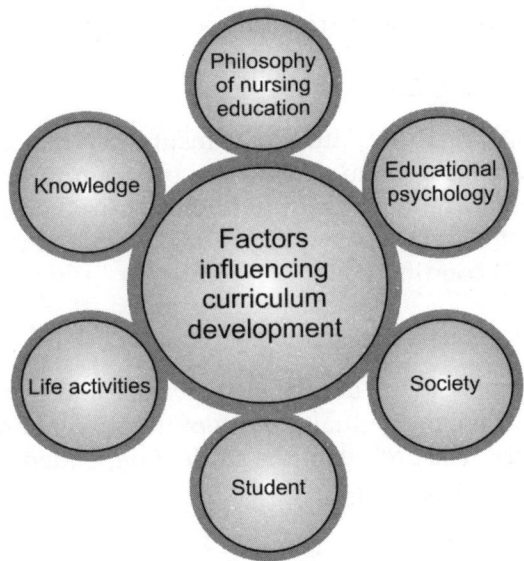

Fig. 28.2: Factors influencing curriculum development

Philosophy of Nursing Education

Philosophy of nursing education is the vital factor in the curriculum. It forms the basis for the final section of the aims and the objectives of the curriculum. Since a major purpose of education is to bring about changes in the behavior of the student, the type of changes to be brought about is one of the most important problems of education. To determine what changes are desired involves value judgments and is influenced by the underlying philosophy of the curriculum.

Educational Psychology

Educational psychology provides the background for the selection of the aims and the objectives of the curriculum.

Educational psychology is the science which provides data and the problems of learning through experimentation. It provides us with data from which the principles of learning are developed. The principles of learning, in turn, provide the basis for the development of principles and methods of teaching. Educational aims and objectives are the educational ends, they have the results to be achieved through learning (to insert from WHO).

Society and Nursing Curriculum

Since the man by nature is the social being, society is nature to man. The social need of man is further met through the educational institutions and the instrument used to meet this need is the curriculum. The relationship between the society and education is 2-way process each influence the other.

Implication for curriculum development: Changes in the family, socioeconomic patterns, political system will influence the curriculum development.

The Student and the Nursing Curriculum

To assist students in adjusting to the educational institutions the curriculum is developed including guidance, counseling, and orientation program to each learning situation. The student is considered as the whole individual to learn and adjust not only by her intellectual capacity but also by her emotional make up, attitude, social relationship and her mental, physical condition.

Life Activities and the Nursing Curriculum

Life activities include professional, family, civic, leisure and spiritual. The curriculum should be focused on for the individual growth of the student and social participation as a citizen of the country. The growth of the student dependent on the factors such as:

1. Changes in the health of the nation
2. Changes in nursing function
3. Changes in nursing education
4. Socioeconomic and political forces
5. Technological forces which negatively influence the learner.

In changing society new function and responsibility have been increasingly added throughout the year. So need analysis will also help in reconstruction of curriculum. The abilities agreed upon by the profession for the practice of nursing can serve as one of the basis for the selection and evaluation of learning experiences.

Knowledge and the Curriculum

Knowledge expansion is central to all curriculum development. Descriptive knowledge refers to facts, laws, theories, principles, etc. Normative knowledge refers to rules, norms, standards by which the individual makes moral or esthetic choices. Knowledge can be organized into specific branches generally referred to as disciplines.

Example:
- General sciences
- Political sciences
- Biological sciences
- Psychosocial sciences
- Nursing science.

Discipline is viewed as "way of learning" and the development of the skills of critical inquiry.

Selection of Learning Experiences in the Curriculum

Since the curriculum has been defined to include all learning experiences planned and guided by the faculty to achieve their stated objectives, the selection of learning experiences which will most likely help to attain those objectives becomes one of the central problems of curriculum planning and development.

Organization of Learning Experiences in the Curriculum

Approaches to Curriculum Organization

After the content knowledge and learning experiences have been selected carefully in relation to the desired objectives, they must be organized in the curriculum. Selection and organization of learning experiences in the curriculum can be grouped under three major approaches. They are: Sociological, Psychological, Logical.

Function of the Organization of the Curricular Elements

The organization of the subject matter content and the learning experiences into an effective, efficient and practical curriculum is very difficult and complex problem, which has received very little attention by educators until recent years. Changes in behavior, in relation to the acquisition of knowledge and the development of skills and attitudes, develop slowly; they are not produced by one single learning experience. In order to produce change, the curriculum should be organized effectively.

Criteria for the Organization of Learning Experiences in the Curriculum

The elements of the curriculum should be related to one another vertically and horizontally so that a systematic body of ideas and activities will be expanded continuously into larger and more meaningful patterns. Criteria which can serve as guides for the effective organization of content or subject matter and learning experiences in the curriculum are continuity and sequence, integration.

Continuity and Sequence

The vertical organization of learning experiences refers to the relationship existing between different levels of the same subject or skills. It is the recurring emphasis in the learners' experiences upon particular elements. This relation is known as continuity. Related to continuity but going beyond. It is the relationship known as sequence.

The importance of planning, and organizing the curriculum so that the most effective continuity and sequence of learning experiences will result are obvious. Curriculum practices in the arrangement of the sequence of learning experiences various widely. However, these practices fall into two groups: in one group, the curriculum includes

the usual subjects of study and the sequence of experiences usually based according to one of the following:
a. Chronological order: places events in succession it terms of time in which they occur
b. Logical order
c. Difficulty: starts with simple to complex.

Integration

- Integration of knowledge, theory and practice.
- Integration of sciences into nursing.
- Integration of General sciences, Political sciences, Biological sciences, Psychosocial sciences, and Nursing sciences.

Core Curriculum

Core curriculum is concerned with the kinds of experiences that will develop the general competencies which all must have in order to live effectively within our democratic way of life.

It emphasis the learning activities that will bring about changing behavior. The core curriculum also include learning experiences that will provide for the development of specialized various types f competencies based on the recognition of individual differences in interest attitudes and capacities. Core curriculum is organized around types of problems of personal and social consent common to all students.

Application of computer skills added in nursing in order to acquire technological competencies for effective management of health care and to be for with scientific advantacement.

As India is multilinguistive country, in every state the state languages are introduced in the curriculum to the nursing student to be competent in their communication skills in order to converse with their clients effectively.

Successful implementation of a core curriculum requires wide range of cooperating planning by teacher and by student teacher planning. For example, students are encouraged to develop skills in preparing their learning objectives.

FACTORS INFLUENCING CURRICULUM CHANGES

1. **Subject matter:** Subject matter is too shallow without addressing the needs, interest, abilities of the students and not encourage in-depth understanding.
2. **Learning experiences:** Learning experiences are arranged based (e.g. medical-surgical nursing) on the hospital classification system of patient rather than any sound educational rationale.
3. **Correlation between theory and clinical practices:** There is minimum or no correlation between the theory learned by the students and clinical practice.
4. **Selection of clinical learning experiences:** There is more concern for meeting service needs of the hospital rather than selecting the clinical learning experiences on the basis of clinical learning objectives.

5. **Application of principles:** Minimal help is given to students in the application of principles from basic discipline to nursing courses and nursing clinical course to clinical practice. The example is the principles of cultural, psychosocial, legal, ethical aspects of care are often forgotten.
6. **Individual learner/students:** Student has fewer roles in making their choices and assuming their responsibility. Often decided by the teacher or administrator.
7. **Learning process:** Less attention is given for systematic learning process.

   The student learn the best when they:
   - Know what their goals are?
   - Are motivated by the relevance of these goals to their personal/professional needs?
   - Work in a small tutorial group.
   - Can alternate between personal study and work in a small tutorial group?
   - Are in an active situation, with responsibilities and a specific objective?
   - Are in a good environment (calm, good staff/student relations, competent, teaching staff, lively atmosphere)?
   - Are able to work at any their own pace?
   - Are able to put what they have learned into their practice (repetition).
   - Learned by the problem based method.
   - Have opportunity for formatting self-evaluation and critical review by others (peer evaluation)?
   - Are exposed to different types of stimulation visual, extended listening, summary review?
   - Face the challenge of valued certifying evaluation.
   - Know that they shall have to inform and instruct others.
   - Are able to have outside contacts (travel, attend conferences, educational tour, etc.) (WHO workshop)?

Preparation of Nursing Curriculum

The nursing curriculum consist of two types of preparation:
1. Foundational
2. Professional
   - The *Foundational* part of the curriculum includes a liberal arts program which leads to the personal development of the student and provides her with principles from the basic disciplines upon which the nursing courses are built.
   - The *Professional* aspects of the curriculum include courses in nursing and related fields. Therefore, the curriculum for the preparation of a nurse who can carry out these professional functions humanely and competently must be developed.

Note

Societal Curriculum

It refers to the syllabus prepared by the statutory bodies such as INC, State Nursing Council, Universities, State Nursing Boards, which is prepared for unifying the curriculum standards throughout the Central and State levels.

For example, Designing of syllabus/Regulations for Post Diploma, MPHW's, GNM, BSc (N), PC BSc (N), MSc (N) and PhD Nursing Programs.

Institutional Curriculum

It refers to the preparation of overall curriculum planning such as Master Plans, Clinical Rotation which will be helpful in implementing the societal curriculum.

Instructional Curriculum

It refers to development of course outlines/course planning in each subject, unit plans and lesson plans which is used for teaching students, each subject in the prescribed hours.

[Examples of master plans, course outlines, unit and lesson plans, clinical rotation plan ... ref. to appendices].

29 Planning and Organization of Clinical Learning Experiences

INTRODUCTION

If you hear you will forget, if you see you remember, if you do it you will learn it (chine's proverb).

So practice is always important followed by a classroom teaching. Before the student is exposed to clinical areas, one needs to practice in the laboratory or demonstration room. The teacher or clinical instructor should demonstrate the procedure how to perform with return demonstration. So that, the student will develop confidence before performing on the client and become competent.

I. General Principles in Selecting Learning Experiences

1. The learning experience must give the student opportunity to deal with the kind of content implied by the objective.
2. The learning experience must be such that the student obtains satisfaction from carrying on the kinds of behavior implied by the objective.
3. The reactions desired in the experience are within the range of possibility for the students involved.
4. There are many particular experiences that can be used to attain the same educational experience.
5. The learning experiences are within an environment that enables the student to complete the assignment given within the time of experience.
6. The learning experiences are structured so that factors which are extraneous to the focus of learning are minimized or eliminated.

II. General Plan for Learning-based on:

1. Objectives to be attained
2. Content of theory
3. Available resources
4. Time element

III. Criteria used in Selecting Clinical Area for Student Experience

1. There are patients present with the kinds of needs which will provide the nursing student with the planned experience.
2. Nursing and medical personnel are cooperative and willing to work with nursing students.

3. The nursing care given to patients is of good quality.
4. The physical facilities and equipment are adequate.

IV. Planning Activities that will Establish Effective Relationships with Staff

1. **Orient them to :**
   a. The objectives of the nursing student's experience.
   b. The educational level of the student.
2. **Ask them about:**
   a. Ward policies.
   b. Nursing procedures peculiar to that clinical area.
3. **Discuss with them:**
   a. The student's role in the nursing team.
   b. The students responsibilities to
      i. The patient
      ii. The head nurse
      iii. The team leader
      iv. The team members
      v. The instructor
   c. Problems they have encountered with different student groups.
   d. Importance and value of their participation in the education of nursing students.
4. **Request of them:**
   a. Permission to orient all wards personnel to the objectives of the student's experience and the role he or she will assume in the nursing team.

V. Planning Students Experiences in Cooperation with the Head Nurse and Team Leaders

1. Review of objectives of experience.
2. Available experiences.
   a. Experiences needed by all students.
   b. Experiences needed by individual students.
3. Assignment of students to nursing team, based upon available experiences.
4. Assignment of students to particular experiences (discuss value of student's choosing own experience.)
5. Review of nursing student's functions and responsibilities.
6. Scheduling of nursing rounds in which head nurse are team leader might participate.
7. Daily appointment with head nurse and team leaders to identify and discuss problems, new learning situations, assignment of experiences, etc.
8. Weekly conference with team leaders to discuss progress of nursing students.
9. Post-nursing students assignment **in advance to allow time for preparation.**

VI. Orientation of Students to Clinical Area

1. Review objectives of the experience (objectives originally structured by the students and instructors).
2. Supplement or revise the objectives as suggested by the students and instructors.
3. Describe methods and responsibilities inherent in:
   a. Assignments
   b. Conferences, rounds, etc.
   c. Evaluation
4. Describes students responsibility as a member of the nursing team to:
   a. Patient/family
   b. Head nurse
   c. Instructor
5. Explain policies and procedures peculiar to the clinical area.
6. Orientation to the personnel, patient, physical facilities and equipment of the clinical area.

VII. Assignments

1. Learning experiences are selected to meet the laboratory focus of the week and thereby correlate classroom theory with clinical practice.
2. Faculties make the assignments in advance of the experience and post the assignments to enable the students to prepare for the experience. Patient identity is not revealed.
3. Faculty may assist each other in making assignments by sharing information and making recommendation.
4. Student needs and request should be kept in mind while making assignments. Students should be encouraged to verbalize interest and needs.
5. Multiple assignments may be of value when the patients needs are complex and/or when a student can benefit from the support and assistance of another student.
6. Procedure for selection of experiences needs to be worked out with staff on the unit. Some suggestions are as follows:
   a. Review lab focus and specific objectives.
   b. Review student needs and request.
   c. Determine level of care, type and amount of care needed by patient assigned to students. Select patients that need care that is appropriate to the level of learning.
   d. Discuss tentative assignments with appropriate staff person.
   e. Complete worksheet with copy for staff, copy for posting and a copy for yourself.
   f. Review charts as necessary to understand patient and his care.
   g. Attend patient report.

ORGANIZING LEARNING EXPERIENCES

- General - Theory
  - Lab — All requirements to be planned in the curriculum.
  - Clinical

Clinical learning experience factors to be considered:
- Learning objectives.
- Level of students, e.g. I year, II year, III year, Interns, etc.
- Background knowledge on theory should posses' adequate relevant theoretical knowledge. Clinical skills – prior exposure to clinical skills whether had opportunity to practice in the laboratory.
- Attitudes and aptitudes of students – self-interest and motivation of students in learning.

Planning of clinical experience: Planning of clinical experience should be based on:
1. Number of students in each clinical area.
2. Availability of patients/opportunity for clinical teaching, e.g. patient : student ratio.
3. Category/classification of patients: dependent, independent and convalescent/ambulatory.
4. Number of staff nurse available – student – staff ratio.

Organization and Implementation of the Plan

1. Assign the patients depending on the background of the students and according to learning objectives.
2. Allocate the no patients depending on the category of patients and individual ability of the students (Strengths and weakness and patient : nurse ratio).
3. Identify and meet the learning needs – what was learnt, yet to learn)
4. Up date the student clinical profile as continuous process.
5. Provide opportunities to meet the objectives of clinical practice, e.g. look out for any rare procedures and help them to practice.
6. Maintain logbook/anecdotal notes to give adequate and equal attention to all students as much as possible.
7. Avoid duplication in assigning patients. For example, assigning the same patients every day or most of the time for same person or changing patient assessment every day which interprets in assessing the care.

Clinical Skill Training

I. Clinical skills are professional tasks to be acquired by a student nurse related to patient care in any health care setting.

   Training is the method of preparation of learners to achieve the ultimate goal or desired clinical learning objectives.

II. Purposes of clinical skill training.
   1. To develop the skills of learner in all the three domains: (a) practical, (b) communication and, (c) intellectual skills.
   2. To develop self-confidence in performing the procedure related to patient care.
   3. To be an efficient nurse-organizing the time and care appropriately.
   4. To deliver patient care effectively–provide patient care as needed according to the priority.

STRATEGIES/METHODS OF CLINICAL TEACHING

Orientation

Learning objectives and evaluation strategies.
- Ward routines
- Patient care policies
- Patient care management
- Ward teaching plans

Demonstration

- Assess the previous knowledge and exposure to performance of a particular procedure, e. g. use of nebulizer for an adult patient.
- Assess the indication and contraindication.
- Involve all the students who did not get opportunity.
- Show or perform the procedure in actual situation or demonstrate well a head of time if time permits.
- Follow the steps of the systematically applying scientific principles (rational).
- After care of the patient and equipment.
- Demonstration–document the time, what procedure is done, and effect of the procedure and response of client to the procedure.
- Return demonstration by the students.

Nurse Rounds and Clinical Rounds

- The nursing rounds are conducted at the bride of client by discuss the relevant patient care management to be performed when students ate new to this experience, e.g. immediate postoperative care of a patient with laparotomy.
- *Clinical rounds* also could help students gain clinical knowledge to understand the progress of the patient and further management.

Pre- and Postconferences

Preconference

At the beginning of the day preconference—briefing of the days plan of work and learning objectives to be achieved by the end of the day need to be discussed and any special programs, planned care study discussions to be informed. This will enable the students to plan and organize themselves to fit into the routines of the wards.

1. Discuss specific objectives.
2. Ascertain student preparedness, appropriateness of attire, and capability to function.
3. Review assignments and discuss new developments, questions/concerns.
4. Establish time for specific supervision or assistance with patient care.
5. Establish time and place of postconference.
6. Review nursing care plans.

Postconference

At end of the day evaluate the days work by revising the student performances, objectives achieved, etc. this will enable the preceptor and the student to be more accountable for teaching and learning.

Objectives

- To "bridge the gap" between nursing theory and the application of theoretical principles in a systematic manner utilizing the nursing process.
- To share experiences with others in order to enhance and reinforce learning.
- To identify common patient problems.
- To make generalizations which might be significant in related patient care situations.
- To provide opportunities for ventilation of feeling if absolutely necessary.
- To provide opportunities to rotate student leadership of group.

Ward Teaching/Case Study Presentation

Ward teaching is an other method by which students can prepare themselves on any aspects of health relevant to their clinical area and conduct the teaching program in the presence of a group of students or staff nurses. This experience will give them opportunity to learn in depth of the aspects of care and gain confidence to develop their oral and written communication, e.g. nursing care of patient with IHD.

Application of Nursing Process

1. Assessment
   a. Identifying Data:
      i. Name
      ii. Diagnosis
      iii. Age
      iv. Religion
      v. Therapy
      vi. Diagnostic measures

2. Identification of needs and problems
   a. Physical
      i. Observable signs and symptoms
      ii. Expressed by patient
      iii. Patients chart
         - History
         - Laboratory findings
   b. Psychosocial
3. Nursing plan and interventions
   a. Reason for nursing action.
   b. Independent or dependent actions.
   c. Scientific principles underlying nursing action.
4. Evaluation of action.
   Outcome criteria.

Components of Clinical/Ward Teaching

- Make rounds to evaluate student progress or difficulty.
- Give direct assistance with patient care in the event of unforeseen development. Return assignment if it is too overwhelming for effective student learning.
- Supervise specific competencies using established critical element checklist.
- Elicit rationale for specific nursing actions from students to evaluate their application of theory to practice.
- Keep staff informed of patient care developments as appropriate to effective communication.
- Make notations of observations of student needs and progress.
- Establish priorities of supervision with consideration of patient needs and students ability to meet needs.
- Use medical and nursing staff as resource people and encourage student collaboration.
- Check charting for accuracy, completeness, etc.
- Have student's record appropriate data on patient care plans.
- Have students report off duty to appropriate person.
- Complete incident reports in conjunction with students and staff.
- Correct nursing care plans and return with comments.
- Unsatisfactory plans must be rewritten.

Ward Staff Meetings

Attending staff meeting organized by ward in-charges at definite intervals will help the team to function effectively and efficiently as the matters related to hospital and patient care policies, and any irregularities observed, issues related to general discipline or achievements, success could be communicated. Wards meeting are essential to maintain the team spirit and interpersonal relationships and quality patient care.

Application of nursing process in the care of an adult patient

Assessment			Planning			Implementation of care		Evaluation of care	
Subjective data	Objective data	Identification of problems/nursing diagnosis	Establish Nsg.goals	Prioritizing intervention	Carry out interventions	Rationale	Outcome criteria	Progress of the client
Client express that he is feeling warm and restless	Temp.38°C Restless mucus membrane is dry Unit is warm	Altered body temperature more than normal. 39°C	To reduce fever maintain normal body temp.	To perform cold application	Cold sponge is given for an hour	Reduces body temp by vasoconstriction and evaporation	Reduce the temp by 2°C at the end of one hr.	Temp. is reduced to 37.2°C by one hr
				To check and administer antipyretics as per prescription	Administered Tab. paracetamol 500 mg as per the prescription	Brings down the temp.	Reduce the temp by 1°C at the end of 1/2 hr.	Temp. is stared reducing to 37.2°C with in 1/2 - one hr
				To monitor body temp. every 2 hrs	Monitored body temp. every 2 hrs	To assess the degree of temp. altered	Continues decline is observed in the body temp. to normal	Fever is reduced gradually
			To prevent dehydration	To encourage to have more fluids	Encouraged to have more fluids as desired	To reduce dehydration and replace body fluids	Normal skin integrity is maintained	Skin and mucus membrane look healthy adequately hydrated maintained normal urinary output Fluids tolerated
				To maintain cool and comfortable environment as tolerated	Maintained cool and comfortable environment as tolerated by Mr. S	To make the client relax and comply with the treatment and care	The unit environment is at the comfort zone	The environment of the unit is cool and comfortable with fans on/Ac, etc. Comfortable clothing
			To reduce to anxiety level and help to relax	To reassure the client with feedback on care given	Reassured the client with feedback on care given and progress	To reduce anxiety and fear	Client feels relaxed	Feels relaxed and able to restwell

Counseling

Individual counseling is an essential component and considered as the best method of teaching a value education and gives an opportunity to listen to their problems of students. The corrective measures are to be given by giving constructive criticisms.

Counseling gives an opportunity to students to introspect themselves, i.e. to identify their strengths and weakness and adapt to alternative methods for self improvement.

Evaluation

i. Anecdotal notes need to be made for each experience and specifically address the students assignment and his/her ability to complete all assigned tasks. Positive and negative comments are recorded with appropriate explanations. Students should be aware of problems/progress and their signature and date will testify to their reading of the comments.

ii. Use an evaluation tool which identifies critical elements of practice.
   a. Make a worksheet with space to check critical elements each clinical day.
      - Document problem areas and discuss with student.
      - Obtain signature to document understanding of problem.
      - Establish goals for improved performance.
      - Establish time expectations.
      - Discuss problems with course faculty to obtain agreement on existence of problem and appropriateness of handling/resolution. Document faculty discussion in minutes of faculty meeting.
      - Involve staff only in unusual cases:
        – Withdraw student from unit
        – Gross violations of policy
        – Partial negligence
        – Gross violation of standards of care.

Evaluation in Education— Qualities of Measuring Instruments

INTRODUCTION

Education is defined as a process developed for bringing about changes in the student's behavior. At the end of a given learning period there should be a greater probability that types of behavior regarded as desirable will appear; other types of behavior regarded as undesirable should disappear.

The educational objectives define the desired types of behavior taken as a whole; the teacher should provide a suitable environment for the student's acquisition of them.

Evaluation in education is a systematic process which enables the extent to which the student has attained the educational objectives always includes measurements (quantitative or qualitative) plus a value judgment.

To make measurements, measuring instruments must be available which satisfy certain requirements so that the results mean something to the teacher himself, the school, the student and society which, in the last analysis, has set up the educational structure.

In education, measuring instruments are generally referred to as "tests".

QUALITIES OF A MEASURING INSTRUMENT—GENERAL

Validity

It is defined as the extent to which the instrument really measures what it is intended to measure. Notion of validity is relative one. It implies a concept of a degree, i.e. very valid; moderately valid; or not valid results. It is also specific to a particular subject.

Content Validity

It is determined by answering the question. Will this test measure or has it measured the matter or behavior indented to measure?

Predictive Validity

Predictive validity is referred to when the results of a tests are to be used for predicting the performance of a student in an other domain or situation.

For example, to what extent results obtained in nutrition and dietetics help to predict the performance in caring for adult patients in adult health nursing.

Reliability

It is defined as the consistency with which an instrument measures a given variable. The instrument is said to be valid when it is relevant and reliable. A question is relevant if it adds to the validity of the instrument. And instrument is relevant if it respects the specifications, i.e. objectives and levels of all three domains of taxonomy and balance of questions. Reliability is a strictly statistical concept.

Objectivity

The extent to which several independent competent examiners agree on what constitutes an acceptable level of performance.

Practicability

The overall simplicity of the use of a test both for test constructor and for a student.

Equilibrium, Equity and Specificity

Instrument is prepared on the basis of objectives and subject content. Examination can be equitable without being valid or relevant if it is not adequately derived from the objectives. Equity and reliability will affect the reliability of the results.

Equilibrium

Achievement of the correct proportion among questions allocated to each of the objectives.

Equity

Extent to which question set in the exam correspond to teaching content.

Specificity

Obtaining a result equivalent to that expected by an intelligent student who in fact has not followed the teaching.

OTHER SPECIFIC QUALITIES OF A MEASURING INSTRUMENT (FIG. 30.1)

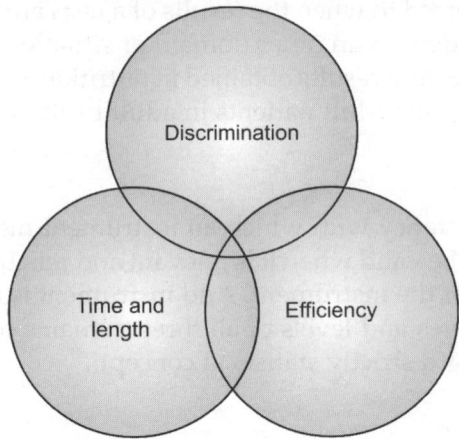

Fig. 30.1: Specific qualities of measuring instruments

Assessment

Assessment is often equated and confused with evaluation, but the two concepts are different.
- Assessment is used to determine what a student knows or can do,
- While evaluation is used to the worth or value of a course or program.

What Questions do you have Regarding Assessment?

- Where do I begin? The first step in designing a quality assessment is to analyze your learning situation by:
  1. Outlining goals and objectives.
  2. Determining the type of learning those outcomes represent (e.g., memorizing concepts, analyzing data, synthesizing resources, etc.).
- What types of test items are available and when should I use them?
  This section outlines pros and cons of different test item types.
- Should I grade my assessments on a bell curve, or is it ok if all my students get "A's"? This section helps differentiate between norm referenced competitive tests and criterion – referenced mastery tests to help you determine the most appropriate purpose for your assessment.
- How can I analyze a completed test to determine its accuracy and effectiveness?
- What testing tools are available to design online quizzes for classroom or group performance.

Analyze Learning Situation

Analyzing your learning situation refers to the microprocess of breaking down a specific course goal into instructional steps and perquisite steps. This process has five specific components:

1. Write a goal
2. Place the goal within a domain of learning
3. List/diagram all steps required to achieve the goal (i.e. instructional analysis)
4. Note prerequisites steps that precede instructional steps
5. Write specific objectives for instructional steps.

Selecting Test Items

You selection of item should be based on the types of outcomes you are trying to assess. Certain item types such as true/dales, supplied response, and matching, work well for lower-order outcomes (i.e. knowledge or comprehension goals), while other item types such as performance assessments, and some multiple choice questions, are better for assessing higher outcomes (i.e. analysis, synthesis, or evaluation goals). A test blueprint specifies your outcome that types of items you plan to use to assess those outcomes.

The table below lists number of explicit behaviors representative of different levels of cognitive thinking. Also listed are common products or outcomes of those behaviors.

	Know remember	*Comprehend understand*	*Use apply*	*Analyze take apart*	*Synthesize create*	*Evaluate judge new*
Behaviors	Name	Describe	Translate	Sort	Design	Rate
	Memorize	Discuss	Practice	Classify	Plan	Value
	Record	Give	Illustrate	Distinguish	Propose	Appraise
	List		Sketch	Experiment	Arrange	Decide
	Match	**Examples**	Solve	Compare	Assemble	Choose
	Write	Locate	Show	Contrast	Develop	Score
	State	Tell	Employ	Diagram	Produce	Select
	Repeat	Find		Debate	Organize	Assess
		Report		Solve	Manage	Debate
		Predict		Examine	Revise	Recommend
		Review		Inventory		
		Recognize				
		Estimate				

31 Test Construction and Item Analysis

INTRODUCTION

An assessment is evidence – gathering procedure for making decisions. The procedure can be formal or informal. Tests are formal assessments which can provide more systematic and objective evidence.

Students assessments can help the teachers understand the following:
- Are students ready for the next learning experience?
- How well the learning goals are met by the students?
- How far are students progressing beyond the minimum?
- What learning problems are students having?
- Which students need to be referred for help?
- Which students have poor insight into their performance?
- What grades should be assigned?
- How effective the teaching was?

The Role of Assessment in the Educational Process

Educational process involves formulation of teaching, learning objectives including all thee domains, the teachers performance of teaching the subject, students performance and the efforts taken by the student in learning, the type of assessments carried out, the results and the feedback.

All these factors reveal the system of education, its strengths and weakness. Suggests for review in the curriculum or the teacher or teaching styles, the process of recruitment of students or improvements to be brought in the infrastructure in the educational institutions.

Assessment and Learning Objectives

The teacher need to think what she wants her student to learn.

Content Issues

Basic knowledge and understanding of specific concepts and techniques.

Process/Skill Issues

- Higher order, critical thinking
- Effective communication in verbal and written
- Working effectively with others

Principles of Classroom Assessment using Tests

- It should be based on understanding how students learn
- Be representative of what was covered in the class
- Accommodate individual differences
- Allow students reflect on learning
- Be clearly explained to students grading criteria
- Be designed to promote further growth
- Be valid and have reliable process
- Allow for timely feedback
- Be an integral part of course development and implementation
- Compose test items as you progress trough the course.

Steps in Developing and using Test

- Determine the outcomes to be measured
- Develop a test blueprint
- Write test items
- Review, critique, and edit the items and proofread
- Obtain reliability and validity data
- Revise, reuse and report.

Blueprint

Blueprint is a plan for constructing the test items based on learning objectives of each subjects. It serves as a guidelines for the teacher to test the level of knowledge acquired by the student in an uniform way. It includes recall, comprehension, analysis and synthesis [refer to appendix for sample].

Types of Test Items

1. Limited choice
2. Open ended.

Limited Choice Items

- Multiple choice questions (MCQs)
- Matching
- True/False

Open Ended

- Sentence completion
- Short answer questions
- Essay questions

Comparison between Limited Choice and Open Ended Questions

Limited choice	Open ended
Sample used more broadly over subject matter	Call for the inclusion of many specifics and tests comprehensiveness.
Faster feedback	Reveal strength and weakness in processing such as comprehension and reasoning.
Fail to foster divergent thinking	Provide more opportunity for creative or divergent thinking comprehension and reasoning.
Give no practice in writing	Provide opportunities for writing.
Favor students who read well	Take longer time.
Are more appropriate for short quizzes	Harder to grade consistently. Reliability can be enhanced by establishing model answers. Working towards inter-rater agreement.
Take more time. Extremely difficult to write good items.	Easier to generate open ended items. Time consuming to grade.
Large number of items is easier to reuse.	Easy to remember and transmit questions to others.
Provide easier conditions for cheating. Can be minimized by using alternate test forms and control seating	Cheating is minimal.

Multiple Choice Items

MCQs can be used in the following situations:
- Analyze phenomena
- Apply principles to new situations
- Comprehend concepts and principles
- Discriminate between fact and opinion
- Interpret cause-effect relationships
- Interpret charts and graphs
- Judge the relevance of information
- Make inferences from given data
- Solve problems.

Which are not ideal to use MCQs:
- Articulate explanations
- Display thought processes
- Furnish information
- Organize personal thoughts
- Perform a specific task
- Produce original ideas
- Provide examples.

An important principle in setting questions one should focus on the "why" and "how" rather than simply asking for factual information.

Teachers should be cautious about tests written by others. Often, items developed by a previous teacher, a textbook author can save a lot of time, but they should be checked for accuracy and appropriateness in the given course.

Test Format–MCQs

- Place similar type of items together to minimize the number of direction needed.
- Place less difficult items at the beginning to make students fell at ease.
- Proofread the test by an other person within or outside the examination committee.
- Balance proportion of correct answers and avoid patterning in the sequencing answers.

For example
Q. Nos: 1   2   3
Ans.   b   c   d

Questions should Test All Three Domains

Bloom's Taxonomy Levels

- Evaluation
- Synthesis
- Analysis
- Application
- Comprehension
- Knowledge

Formulation of Questions

The following are the examples used to construct the stem of the questions.
- Knowledge questions: the stem of questions include – define, lable, list, describe, name, etc.
- Comprehension- Explain discusses, indicate, locate application – apply, choose, solve, illustrate, identify, predict, paraphrase, etc.
- Analysis- compare, contrast, distinguish, differentiate, etc.
- Synthesis- formulates, construct, create, arrange, etc.
- Evaluation- appraise, evaluate, judge, estimate, etc.

Levels of Test Construction—MCQs

Level 1: Knowledge

It deals with the recall of acquired knowledge.

Example: Night blindness is deficiency of which of the following vitamins?
a. Vitamin A
b. Vitamin B
c. Vitamin C
d. Vitamin D

Level 2: Comprehension

At this level knowledge of facts, theories, procedures, etc. is assumed and one should test for understanding of this knowledge.

Example: If you find the physicians order on drug sheet as Tab. Paracetamol for fever "p r n" and client experiences no reduction in fever "what should you do"?

In this question, the knowledge of the various section must be recalled (knowledge) and understanding (comprehension) meaning of each term.

Level 3: Application

Application to the situation need to be understood while answering the question.

Example: Nurse Sharon is assigned to care for Mr. Colin 57 years, who was admitted with the complaints of severe diarrhea, vomiting abdominal cramps and fever.

Which of the following actions is the most appropriate to relieve Colins abdominal cramps.

Note: In order to answer this question relevant actions/interventions should be known and understood. It means evaluation of given situation is necessary.

Four relevant options are required to stimulate creative thinking and analysis of a given situation.

Level 4: Synthesis: Formulates, construct, create, arrange, etc.

Level 5: Evaluation: Appraise, evaluate, judge, estimate, etc.

Qualities of a Test

- Directly related to educational objectives
- Realistic and practical
- Concerned with important and useful matters
- Comprehensive but brief
- Precise and clear.

Common Defects of Examinations (Domain of intellectual skills)

1. Triviality
2. Outright error
3. Ambiguity
4. Obsolescence

5. Bias
6. Complexity
7. Unintended cues

Outside Factors to be Avoided

1. Complicated instructions (ability to understand instructions)
2. Over-elaborate style (ability to avoid traps)
3. Trap questions (ability to use words)
4. "Test-wise"

Essay examinations

Advantages	Disadvantages
1. Provide candidate with opportunity to demonstrate his knowledge and his ability to organize ideas and express them effectively.	1. Limit severely the area of the student's total work that can be sampled 2. Lack objectivity 3. Provide little useful feedback 4. Take a long time to score

Multiple choice questions

Advantages	Disadvantages
1. Ensure objectivity, reliability and validity; preparation of questions with colleagues provides constructive criticism 2. Increase significantly the range and variety of facts that can be sampled in a given time 3. Provide precise and unambiguous measurement of the higher intellectual processes 4. Provide detailed feedback for both student and teachers 5. Are easy and rapid to score	1. Take a long time to construct in order to avoid arbitrary and ambiguous questions 2. Also require careful preparation to avoid preponderance of questions testing only recall 3. Provide cues that do not exist in practice 4. Are "costly" where number of students is small

ITEM ANALYSIS

After a test is administered. It is necessary to judge the quality of test items particularly in limited - choice test. It helps in quality control over the type of questions used especially when there is a plan to retain them for reuse. Well specified objectives and well constructed items give you a head start in the process, but item analysis gives you feedback on how successful you actually were.

The factors which affect the quality of measuring instrument:
- Reliability
- Discrimination
- Length

- Homogeneity of questions
- Heterogeneity of students.

Reliability is influenced by the extend to which the items in the test paper clearly distinguish competent from incompetent students.

The number of items and the similarity of the items as regards their power to measure a given skill and the extend to which the students are not similar with respect to that skill.

The level of its difficulty directly influences the discriminating power of a question, and heterogeneity of the students.

The discrimination index of a test is also affected by the homogeneity of the question and heterogeneity of the students.

Equity will also influence the discriminating power of the test.

Methods to Measure Reliability

- Test–Retest with the same form
- Use two equivalent forms of a test
- Derive two scores from the same test. Split – half test

Reliability coefficient (r) is calculated as:

$$r = \frac{1 - M(K - M)}{K\sigma^2}$$

Where M = mean of the test score
 K = no. of items in the test
 σ^2 = Variance (Squared sd) Standard squared deviation score.

For a GOOD TEST "r" should be at least 0.6.
If 'r' < 0.6 then to reach 'r' = 0.6 we do item analysis
Reliability is : – 1 to + 1.

Purposes of Item Analysis

It helps to identify:
a. How effective is a given item in a total test paper?
b. Discover functionally good/poor items.
c. Isolate the reason for poor construction of test items and revise for next use.
d. Improve item writing capability.
e. Feedback on capability.
f. It gives information on items difficulty, discriminating power and pattern of response.

Steps for Item Analysis of a Single Test – MCQ Items

a. Correct the test and award a score for each student.
b. Rank the students in the order of merit from the highest to lowest.

c. Identify the highest 33 percent and the lowest 33 percent of the students. Some literature recommend first 27 percent and the last 27 percent or 25 percent or 33 percent.
d. Calculate the difficulty index and discriminating index of a question.
e. Interpret the result and critically evaluate each question to decide whether to retain, reject or revise the items.

Formula and Interpretation of Indexes

Difficulty index refers to means of measuring the easiness or difficulty of a test question. It is the percentage of students who have correctly answered test questions. It would be more logical to call it as easiness index. It can vary from 0 to 100 percent.

Calculation

$$\text{Difficulty index} = \frac{H + L}{N} \times 100$$

Where H = Number of correct answers in the high group
L = Number of correct answers in the low group
N = Total number of students in both groups

Interpretation

The higher the index the easier the question. In principle, a question with a difficulty index lying between 30 and 70 percent is acceptable.

Example:

Result	Meaning	Action
< 30%	The item is hard	Review and change
30 to 70%	The item is good	Retain the item
>70%	The item is too easy	Review and change

If the indexes are in the range of 30 to 70 percent, then the mean index will be around 50 percent. It has been shown that a test with difficulty index in the range of 50 to 60 percent is very likely to be reliable as regards its internal consistency and homogeneity.

Discrimination Index

It is an indicator showing how significantly a question discriminates between the high and low students. It varies from − 1 to + 1; If all upper group got it right and all lower group got it wrong = 100 percent = + 1.

Calculation

$$\text{Discrimination index} = 2 \times \frac{H - L}{N}$$

Where   H = Number of correct answers in high group
L = Number of correct answers in low group
N = Total Number of students in both groups

Interpretation

The higher the index the more a question will distinguish between high and low students in a given group.

Result	Meaning	Action
Negative	More poor questions than good were correct	Discard or change
< 0.15	Both groups did equally well in this item- poor questions	Discard or change
0.15 – 0.24	Some discrimination observed marginal questions	Revise
0.25 – 0.34	Good questions- Item discriminates between groups	Retain the test item (question)
> 0.35	Excellent item. Discriminates between the groups	Retain the test item

When a test is composed with high discrimination indexes it ensures a ranking that clearly discriminates between the students according to their level of performance. It helps to identify who are the best students objectively.

It is useful in preparing question bank. The index serves as indicative rather than absolute value.

Appendices

Appendix 1: Example of master plans

Class: BSc N. I year: Dates: From: to:

Sl. no.	Subjects	Recommended theory		Planned theory		Recommended clinical		Planned clinical		Remarks/other activities
		Hrs/wk	Total hrs	Hrs/wk	Total hrs	Hrs/wk	Total hrs	Hrs/wk	Total hrs	
1.	Basic principles and practice of nursing									Schedule of
2.	Anatomy									• Unit tests
3.	Physiology and biochemistry									• Term exams
4.	Microbiology									• University exams
5.	Psychology									• Clinical postings
6.	Sociology									
7.	English									

- Vacation: No: wks/yr; Dates:
- National holidays/year
- Study holidays/year

Signature of the coordinator   Signature of the Principal/Dean

Date: Date:

Appendix 1A: Master plans

Class: BSc N. II year: Dates: From: to:

Sl. no.	Subjects	Recommended theory		Planned theory		Recommended Clinical		Planned clinical		Remarks/other activities
		Hrs/wk	Total hrs	Hrs/wk	Total hrs	Hrs/wk	Total hrs	Hrs/wk	Total hrs	
1.										Schedule of
2.										• Unit tests
3.										• Term exams
4.										• University exams
5.										• Clinical postings
6.										
7.										

- Vacation: No: Wks/yr; Dates:
- National holidays/year
- Study holidays/year

Signature of the coordinator   Signature of the Principal/Dean

Date: Date:

Appendix 1B: Master plans

Class: BSc N. III year: Dates: From: to:

Sl. no.	Subjects	Recommended theory		Planned theory		Recommended Clinical		Planned clinical		Remarks/other activities
		Hrs/wk	Total hrs	Hrs/wk	Total hrs	Hrs/wk	Total hrs	Hrs/wk	Total hrs	
1.										Schedule of
2.										• Unit tests
3.										• Term exams
4.										• University exams
5.										• Clinical postings
6.										
7.										

- Vacation: No: Wks/yr; Dates:
- National holidays/year
- Study holidays/year

Signature of the coordinator   Signature of the Principal/Dean

Date: Date:

Appendix 1C: Master plans

Class: BSc N. IV year: Dates: From: to:

Sl. no.	Subjects	Recommended theory		Planned theory		Recommended clinical		Planned clinical		Remarks/other activities
		Hrs/wk	Total hrs	Hrs/wk	Total hrs	Hrs/wk	Total hrs	Hrs/wk	Total hrs	
1.										Schedule of
2.										• Unit tests
3.										• Term exams
4.										• University exams
5.										• Clinical postings
6.										
7.										

- Vacation: No: wks/yr; Dates:
- National holidays/year
- Study holidays/year

Signature of the coordinator   Signature of the Principal/Dean

Date: Date:

Appendix 2: Example of clinical rotation plan

Class: III yr BSc Nursing   Dates: From :............. to:.................

Groups

Number of weeks

Groups	1	2	3	4	5	6	7	8	9	10	11	12	13	14	15	16	17	18	19	20	21	22	23	24	25	26	27	28	29	30
I.	Medial ward							Surgical ward						OBG/Maternity						Pediatric ward						Psychiatry ward				
II.	Surgical ward							OBG/Maternity						Pediatric ward						Psychiatry ward						Medial ward				
III.	OBG/Maternity							Pediatric ward						Psychiatry ward						Medial ward						Surgical ward				
IV.	Pediatric ward							Psychiatry ward						Medial ward						Surgical ward						OBG/Maternity				
V.	Psychiatry ward							Medial ward						Surgical ward						OBG/Maternity						Pediatric ward				

Clinical Postings	Duration	Clinical Requirements	Clinical Supervision
Medical and Surgical	6 weeks	Case studies	Teachers concern for each area
OBG / Maternity	6 weeks	Group projects	
Pediatric ward	6 weeks	Procedures required	
Psychiatry ward	6 weeks	Patient education	
		Clinical presentation	

Clinical days : Mon to Sat/week   Timings: 8 am to 1 pm   Clinical Examination Dates: Internal:
                                                                                  External:

Signature of the Coordinator: Signature of the principal:
Date :   Date:

Appendix 3: Example – course plan

Class: III year BSc N
Subject: Child Health Nursing
Total no of Hrs theory: 80 hrs
Lab hrs: 40 hrs
Clinical hrs: 360 hrs

Dates: October 2007 - May 2008
No of weeks:

Week/Dates	Units	Content/chapters	Method of teaching/Learning	Hrs	Evaluation
Wk I	I 5 hrs	Ch 1	Quiz	1	Small tests
		Ch 2	Lecture and Discussion with PPT	2	
Wk II	II 4 hrs	Ch 3	" "	2	Assignments
		Ch 4	" use models "	2	
		Ch 5	" "charts	1	Group work, etc.
		Ch 6	" "PPT	1	
	Lab Session	1	Video/Demonstration of assessment of an Infant	2	Assess an infant and write the findings.

Signature of the Teacher

Date

Signature of the Principal/Dean

Appendix 4: Example of unit plan

Class: BSc N III yr
Course: Pediatric nursing
Unit 1: Introduction to child health nursing
Total no of hrs: 5 hrs

Units	Content	Objectives	Hrs/chapter	T/L activities	Method of Evaluation
I 5 hrs	Chapter 1. Definition, Concepts, principles	Explain the concepts and principles of G and D	1 hr	Discussion	Quiz -15 mts
	Chapter 2. Trends in child health nursing	Discuss and explain about trends in child health nursing	2 hrs	PPT presentation	Assignment on trends in other countries
	Chapter 3. Factors affecting Growth and development	Identify factors influencing G and D	2 hrs	Lecture and discussion	Group work on observations made at home on the child rearing practices, etc.
II	-	-	-	-	-

Signature of the Teacher
Date:

Appendix 5: Example of lesson plan

Class   : III yr BSc (N)
Course   : Introduction to Child Health Nursing
Unit   : 2   Chapter : 2   Topic: Principles of growth and development
Date   : 02-02-2008   Time   : 1 Hour: 9–10 am
Method of Teaching : Lecture and discussion
A-V Aids used   : PowerPoint presentation
Objectives   : Formulate objectives for the class session
Introduction   : Introduce to the class, review previous class and begin with what they know.

Sl. No.	Teaching/learning objectives	Subject content	Teaching/learning activities	Evaluation/feedback
1.				
2.				
3.				
4.				
5.				

Summary/Conclusion :
Assignments: Date of submission: Total Marks:
Bibliography:
Signature of the Teacher:
Date:

Appendix 6: Application of nursing process in the care of an adult patient

Assessment		Planning			Implementation of care		Evaluation of care	
Subjective data	Objective data	Identification of problems/nursing diagnosis	Establish nsg. goals	Prioritizing intervention	Carry out interventions	Rationale	Outcome criteria	Progress of the client
Client express that he is feeling warm and restless	Temp. 38°C Restless mucus membrane is dry unit is warm	Altered body temperature more than normal 39°C	To reduce fever maintain normal body temp.	To perform cold application	Cold sponge is given for an hour	Reduces body temp. by vasoconstriction and evaporation	Reduce the temp. by 2°C at the end of one hr	Temp. is reduced to 37.2°C by one hr
				To check and administer antipyretics as per the prescription	Administered Tab. paracetamol 500 mg as per the prescription	Brings down the temp.	Reduce the temp. by 1°C at the end of 1/2 hr	Temp. is stared reducing to 37.2°C with in 1/2 - one hr
			To prevent dehydration	To monitor body temp. every 2 hrs	monitored body temp. every 2 hrs	To assess the degree of temp altered	Continues decline is observed in the body temp to normal	Fever is reduced gradually
				To encourage to have more fluids	Encouraged to have more fluids as desired	To reduce dehydration and replace body fluids	Normal skin integrity is maintained	Skin and mucus membrane look healthy adequately maintained normal urinary output fluids tolerated
			To reduce to anxiety level and help to relax	To maintain cool and comfortable environment as tolerated	Maintained cool and comfortable environment as tolerated by Mr. S	To make the client relax and comply with the treatment and care	The unit environment is at the comfort zone	The environment of the unit is cool and comfortable with fans on/Ac, etc. comfortable clothing
				To reassure the client with feedback on care given	Reassured the client with feedback on care given and progress	To reduce anxiety and fear	Client feels relaxed	Feels relaxed and able to restwell

Appendix 7: Example of Blue print - Obs. and Gyne Course

Date: 31.12.2007 **Time:** 2½ Hours **Max Marks:** 80 Marks
No. of Test Items: **MCQ:** 32 Marks **Matching:** 8 Marks **Short Answers:** 40 Marks

Units, Objectives, Major Concepts and Time				Level of Learning		Points, Item type and Weightage			
Unit	Objectives	Concepts	Time	Lower (32M) 40%	Higher (48M) 60%	Points	Item	Total	%
I Class Session 1-9	Nursing care of women in normal pregnancy	• History and trends • Anatomy and physiology of female and male reproductive system • Fertilization and fetal development • Placenta, umbilical cord, amniotic fluid and fetal circulation • Physiological changes during pregnancy • Signs and symptoms and diagnosis of pregnancy • Care of women during antenatal period • Nursing care of women with minor disorders	(10 Hrs) 1 hr 2 hrs 1 hr 1 hr 1hr 1 hr 2 hrs 1 hr	1 2 1 1 1 (6 M)	 2 2 4 (8 M)	1 2 1 1 2 2 4	MCQ SA	14	17.5
II Class Session 10-11	Nursing care of women in normal labor	• Nursing care of women in I, II and III stage of labor • Nursing care of women in IV stage of labor and newborn care	(4 Hrs) 2 hrs 2 hrs	1 1 (2 M)	2 2 (4 M)	3 3	MCQ SA	6	7.5
III Class Session 12-15	Nursing care in normal puerperium and newborn	• Physiology and management of puerperium • Physiology of lactation • Family planning concepts and methods • Physiology of newborn, assessment and care of the newborn with minor disorders	(8Hrs) 2 hrs 1 hr 3 hrs 2 hrs	1 1 2 (4 M)	3 4 (7 M)	4 1 2 4	MCQ Matching SA	11	13.75

Contd...

Units, Objectives, Major Concepts and Time				Level of Learning		Points, Item type and Weightage			
Unit	Objectives	Concepts	Time	Lower (32M)	Higher (48M)	Points	Item	Total	%
IV Class Session 16-24	Nursing care of women with high risk pregnancy	• Risk approach and hyperemesis gravidarum • Anemia, heart disease and Infections • Pregnancy induced hypertension • Bleeding in early pregnancy • Antepartum hemorrhage • Multiple pregnancy	(8Hrs) 1 3 1 1 1 1	1 1 1 1 (4 M)	1 4 2 (7 M)	1 5 1 3 1	MCQ Matching SA	11	13.75
V Class Session 26-29	Nursing care of women with complications of labor	• Malpositions and presentations • Induction • Instrumental delivery and caesarian section • Obstetrical emergencies	(6 Hrs) 2 1 1 2	1 1 1 (3 M)	2 3 (5 M)	3 1 4	MCQ SA	8	10
VI Class Session 30-31	Nursing care of women with complications of puerperium	• Postpartum hemorrhage • Puerperal infections	(4 Hrs) 2 2	1 1 (2 M)	2 2 (4 M)	3 3	MCQ SA	6	7.5
VII Class Session 32-35	Nursing care of high-risk new-born babies	• Low birth the weight babies • Asphyxia neonatorum • Neonatal jaundice • Common infections and birth injuries	(4 Hrs) 1 1 1 1	1 1 (2 M)	4 (4 M)	1 1 4	MCQ Matching	6	7.5

Contd...

Units, Objectives, Major Concepts and Time				Level of Learning		Points, Item type and Weightage			
Unit	Objectives	Concepts	Time	Lower (32M)	Higher (48M)	Points	Item	Total	%
VIII Class Session 36-44	Nursing care of women with gynecological disorders		**(13 Hrs)**						
		• Principles and common investigations	1 hr	1		1	MCQ		
		• Care of women with menstrual dysfunction and menopause	2 hrs		4	4	SA		
		• Benign lesions and endometriosis	2 hrs	1	2	3	MCQ		
		• Fistulas and urinary incontinence	2 hrs	1	2	3	MCQ		
		• Genital displacement	1 hr	1		1	MCQ		
		• Malignant disorders of female reproductive system	1 hr	1		1	MCQ	18	22.5
		• Care of women with hysterectomy	1 hr		3	3	SA		
		• Pelvic inflammatory diseases	1 hr	1		1	MCQ		
		• Infertility and management	2 hrs	1		1	MCQ		
				(7 M)	(11 M)				
				30 M (40 %)	50 M (60 %)			80	100

Glossary

Accreditation: An official approval given by an organization stating that it has achieved a required standard.

Accountability: A person is responsible for his/her own actions and decisions and expected to explain them when asked. Being accountable or responsible for the moral and legal requirements of proper patient care.

Autocracy: A country or a system of government of a country which is ruled by one person who has complete power.

Autocrat: A person or a ruler who has complete power and expects to be obeyed by other people and does not care for their opinions or feelings.

Authority: The power to give orders to people. In an organization people who have power to make decisions or who have particular area of in country or region responsibility.

Authoritarian: A leader who believes that the people should obey authority and rules even if they are unfair and even if it means that they loose their personal freedom.

Blueprint: A plan which shows what can be achieved and how it can be achieved.

Body language: The process of communicating what you are feeling and thinking by the way you place and move your body rather than by words.

Bureaucracy: The system of official rules and ways of doing things that a government or an organization has and it seems too complicated.

Bureaucrat: An official working in an organization or government department and specially one who follows the rules too strictly.

Budget: The money that is available to a person or to an organization and a plan of how it will be spent monthly or yearly or defense budget, railway budget, etc.

Charisma: The powerful personal quality that some people have to attract and impress other people.

Communication: It is an activity or process of expressing ideas, feelings or of giving people information.

Commitment: A thing that you have promised or agreed to do so. The willingness to work hard and give your energy and time to a job or an activity.

Command: An order given to a person to carry out a job or an activity.

Control: The power to make decisions about a country, an area, an organization, etc.

Concepts: An idea or principle which connected with a subject.

Contingency: An event which may or may not happen. We must consider all possible.

Contingencies: Contingency plan; plan for what to do if a particular event happens or doesn't happen.

Coordination: To organize the different parts of an activity and the people involved in it. So that it works well.

Cost: The total amount of money that needs to be spent by an organization or a person or government.

Cost-benefit analysis (CBA): A type of economic evaluation of medical care expense, it compares the monitory benefit derived from different health intervention with the cost of providing each of the interventions.

Cost control: The process of monitoring and regulating the expenditure of funds by an agency or institution.

Curriculum: The subjects that are included in a course of a study or taught in a school or a college.

Course plan: A series of lessons or lectures planned on a particular subject.

Decentralization: To give some of the power of a Central Government, organization, etc. to smaller parts or organization around the country.

Decision: A choice or judgment you make after thinking and talking about what is the best thing to do.

Decision making: The process of deciding about something important, especially in a group of people or in an organization.

Democratic: A country or a state a system controlled by representatives who are elected by the people of the country. Based on the principle that all people have are equal right to be involved in running an organization.

Discriminating: Able to judge the good quality.

Effective: Producing the result that is wanted or intended, producing a successful result.

Efficiency: The quality of doing something well with no wastage of time or money.

Ethics: Moral principles that control or influence a person's behavior, e.g. code of ethics. It is a branch of philosophy that deals with moral principles.

Evaluation: To found and opinion of the amount, value or quality of something after thinking about it carefully.

Evidence: The facts, signs or objects that make you believe that is true.

Facilitate: To make an action or a process possible or easier.

Fiscal year: Refers to financial year.

Group dynamics: Work done by a group of people working together.

Healthcare industries: The complex of preventive remedial and therapeutic services provided by hospitals and other institution.

Integrated approach: The act or process of combing two or more things so that they worked together. In which many different parts are closely connected and work successfully together.

Item analysis: To judge the quality of test items particularly in limited-choice test. It helps in quality control over the type of questions used especially when there is a plan to retain them for reuse.

Issues: The most important part of the subject that is being discussed or arguing about.

Job description: A written description of the exact work and responsibilities of a job.

Know-How: Knowledge of how to do a thing and experience a doing it.

Leader: A person who leads a group of people especially the head of the country or organization.

Leadership: The state or position of being a leader.

Logical: An action or events, etc. seeming natural, reasonable or sensible able to follow the rules of logic in which ideas of facts are based on other true ideas or facts.

Management: The act of running or controlling the business or organization.

Manager: A person who is in charge of running business or organization.

Master plans: A detailed plan that will make a complicated project successful.

Mission statement: An official statement of the aims of a company or organization.

Models: A simple description of a system used for explaining how it works or calculating what might happen. A system that can be copied by other people.

Motivation: A person does he what to do by self-interest which involves hard work and interest.

Novice: A person who is new and has little experience in a skill, a job, or situation.

Nursing audit: A thorough investigation designed to identify, examine, or verify the performance of certain specified aspects of nursing care using established criteria.

Nursing Director: A nurse whose function the administrative and clinical leadership of the nursing service of a division of health care facility.

Objectives: Something that you are trying to achieve.

Organization: A group of people who form a business, club, etc. together in order to achieve a particular aim.

Organizational charts: A diagram showing the structure of an organization showing the relationships between all the jobs in it.

Permissive: Allowing or showing a freedom of behavior that many people do not approve of.

Philosophy: A particular set or system of beliefs resulting from the search for knowledge about life or universe.

Plan: Something you intend to do or achieve.

Policy: A plan of action agreed and a principle that you believe in that influences how you behave.

Practice: Action rather than ideas.

Principles: A moral rule or a strong belief that influences your action.

Procedures: The correct way of doing things. The sequence of steps to be followed in establishing some course of action.

Program: A plan of things that will be done or included.

Quality assurance: The practice of managing the way goods are produced or to make sure that they are of high standard.

Quality monitoring: It is a systematic collection and analysis of organizations quality indicators for the purpose of improving patient care.

Reliability: The extent to which a test measurement or device produces the same results with different investigators, observers, or administration of the test overtime.

Responsibility: A duty to deal with or take care of because of your job or position.

Role: The function or position that some one has or expected to have in an organization, in a society or in a relationship.

Roster: A list of people's names and the jobs that they have to do at a particular time. Duty roster is a list of the names of people who are available to do a job at particular time.

Schedule: A plan that list all the work that you have to do and when must do each thing. For example, time table. To arrange things to happen at a particular time.

Standards: A level of quality, especially one that people think is acceptable.

Strategic planning: A plan that is intended to achieve a particular purpose.

Supervision: To be in-charge something and make sure everything is done correctly and safely.

Theories: A formal set of ideas that is intended to explain why something happen or exist.

Trends: A general directions in which a situation is changing or developing.

Unit: A group of people live together for a particular purpose in a hospital or a department that provides a particular type of care or treatment, e.g. Nursing unit.

Validity: A state of being legally or officially acceptable. The extent to which a test measurement or other device measures what it is intended to measure.

Valuation: A professional judgment about how useful or important something and its estimated important.

Weekly schedule: Any work that is planned by week. For example, Time tables or operation list or OT list.

Work force: All the people who work for a particular company or organization.

Work: To do something that involves physical or mental effort as a part of a job.

Work load: Amount of work that has to be done by a particular person or organization.

X-ray: A type of radiation that can pass through the objects that are not transparent and make it possible to see inside. X-ray department or radiology department is an essential diagnostics required for a hospital.

Yearly: Once in a year some work will be planned in an organization. For example, Annual leave plan, annual budget of the department, etc.

Index

A
Appraisal interview 111

B
Blue print–obs. and gyne course 200
Budgeting 62
    budgeting and nursing 62
    objectives 62
    purpose 63
    types 63
        capital budget 64
        operating budget 64
        personnel budget 63

C
Census record 136
Classification of hospitals 75
    administration, ownership, control or financial income 75
        governmental or public hospital 75
        non-governmental or private 75
    length of stay 75
        short-term or short-stay hospitals 75
    size or bed capacity 76
    type of service 75
        general hospitals 75
        special hospitals 75
    types of medical staff 76
        closed-staff hospital 76
        open-staff hospital 76
Clinical rotation plan 195
Common leadership traits 23
Communication 43
    channels of managerial communications 46
        diagonal communication 48
        downward communication 46
        lateral communication 47
        upward communication 47
    communication model 44
    importance 46
    levels of communication 44
        interpersonal communication 44
        intrapersonal communication 44
        mass communication 44
        organizational communication 44
        public communication 44
        small group communication 44
    objectives 43
    types 48
        non-verbal communication 48
        verbal communication 48
Comparison of leadership styles 33
Continuing education program 122
    objectives 122
Control 124
    purpose 124
    types 125
        concurrent control 125
        feedback control 125
Cost benefit analyses 64
Course plan 196
Critical thinking in communication 48
Curriculum planning 160
    criteria 165
        continuity and sequence 165
        integration 166
    factors influence curriculum development 162
        educational psychology 163
        knowledge and the curriculum 164
        life activities and the nursing curriculum 164
        philosophy of nursing education 163
        society and nursing curriculum 164
        student and the nursing curriculum 164
    function 165
    levels 161
        institutional curriculum 162
        instructional curriculum 162
        societal curriculum 161
    organization 165
    selection 165

D
Decision-making and problem solving 59
    advantages 59
    objectives 59
    similarities 59
    steps 60
Development of program objective 149
Differences between the leader and the manager 4

Discrimination index 189
Domain of intellectual skills 186

E

Effective leadership style 33
Essential areas and facilities in the nursing unit 86
    closets 86
    nurse's station 86
    patient rooms 86
Ethics in managing health care 131
    manager's obligation 131
    objective 131
    principles of biomedical ethics 132
Evaluating effectiveness of educational programs 152

F

Factors influencing curriculum changes 166
    application of principles 167
    correlation between theory and clinical practices 166
    individual learner 167
    learning experiences 166
    learning process 167
    selection of clinical learning experiences 166
    subject matter 166
First-line nurse manager (head nurse) 91
    nursing unit management 95
    patient care management 91
        principles of assignment 91
        purpose 91
        types of assignments 92
    staff management 93
        staff development 94
        staff evaluation 94
        staff supervision 94
        staff utilization 94
First-line nurse manager's role 145
    objectives 145
Fluid balance chart 136
    contents 136
Formula and interpretation of indexes 189
Functions of a leader 35

G

Group dynamics 50
    group size 51
    objectives 50
    phases of group dynamics 50
        dependent phase 50
        independent phase 51
        interdependent phase 51
        termination phase 51
    types of groups 50
        formal work groups 50
        informal or social group 50

H

Herzberg's motivation 114
Hospital departments 74
    functions 74
        patient care 74
        health personnel education 74
        health promotion 74
        health related research 74
    objectives 74

I

Integrative leadership model 27
Issues in nursing curriculum development 157
    phases 158
        development phase 158
        evaluation phase 158
        implementation phase 158
        initiation phase 158
Item analysis 187
    purposes 188
    steps 188

J

Job description 106
    information 106
    objectives 106
    purposes of preparing job description in the organization 107
    guidelines for writing job description 107

K

Knowledge 26
    types 26
        knowing business 26
        knowing oneself 26
        knowing organization 26
        knowing the job 26
        knowing the world 26

L

Leadership and management 3
    concepts 4
        general concepts 4
        specific concepts 5
    objectives 3
    primary purpose 3
Leadership and management development 122
    objectives 122
Leadership of a nurse manager 34

Leadership styles 29
   autocratic leadership 30
      advantages 31
      disadvantages 31
   bureaucratic style of leadership 33
   democratic leadership 31
      advantages 32
      disadvantages 32
   laissez-faire leadership 32
      advantages 33
      characteristic features 32
      disadvantages 33
Leadership theories 21
   charismatic theory 21
      Conger and Kanungo's research findings 22
      House's research findings 22
   contingency theory 25
   great man theory 21
   path goal theory 25
   situational theory 24
   trait theory 22
      communication 24
      creative 24
      emotional maturity with integrity 24
      initiative 24
      intelligence 23
      persuasion 24
Lesson plan 198
Line-staff organization 73

M

Management process 8
  nursing management 7
      controlling 10
      directing 9
      organizing 9
      planning 9
      staffing 9
Management theories 11
   behavioral science theory 16
      Likert's theory 18
      McGregor's theory 17
   classic organization theory 13
      Fayol theory 14
      James Mooney theory 15
      Max Webber theory 14
   human relations theory 15
      Follett theory 15
      Lewin theory 16

   objectives 11
   scientific management 12
      Emerson's theory 13
      Gantt theory 12
      Taylor's theory 12
McClelland's basic needs theory 114

N

Narcotic record 136
Non-professional health service departments 80
   accounts (business office) 81
   admitting department 80
   central sterile supply department (CSSD) 82
      purpose 82
   housekeeping department (domestic services) 81
   laundry department 81
   maintenance department 81
   mechanical department 81
   medical records 81
   personnel department (functions) 80
   purchase department 81
   social service department/public relation department 82
      class exercise 82
      purpose 82
      directions 82
      exercise to students 82
Nursing care delivery system 83
   classification of nursing practice personnel 83
      non-professional nursing personnel 84
      professional nursing personnel 83
   function of the nursing department 84
   nursing practice department 83
   objectives 83
Nursing care plan 135
   contents 136
   purposes 135
Nursing information sheet or records 135
   contents 135
   purpose 135
Nursing process in the care of an adult patient 199
Nursing progress sheet 135
   contents 135
   purposes 135
Nursing services standards 96
Nursing unit records 133
   types 133
Nursing unit/ward 84
   specific functions 84

    type of nursing units 85
        general units 85
        nursing unit environment 86
        unit organization 85

O

Objectives of professional education 150
Organization charts 72
    advantages 72
    limitations 73
    principles 72
    types 72
        horizontal charts 72
        vertical charts 72
Organization of the hospital 76
Organizational models 71
Organizational structure 70
    dimensions 71
    importance 70
    objectives 70
    types 71
        formal organization 71
        informal organization 71
Organizing learning experience 152, 172

P

Patient classification system 87
    factor evaluation system 87
    importance 87
    objectives 87
    purpose 87
    types 87
        diagnostic related groups 87
        factor evaluation system 87
        prototype evaluation system 87
Patient's chart 134
    contents 134
    purposes 134
Performance appraisal 108
    characteristics of evaluation tool 110
        objectivity 110
        reliability 110
        validity 110
    evaluation tools 110
        check-list 110
        critical incident technique 111
        essay 111
        faced choice rating 110
        management by objective 111
        peer-review 111
        rating scale 110
        state nursing competencies rating scale 111
    objectives 108
    principles of evaluation 109
    problems in performance appraisal 110
    qualities of evaluation 109
        capacity of further development 109
        mental qualities 109
        personnel qualities 109
        quality of performance 109
        supervisory qualities 109
    staff evaluation tools and techniques 110
Planned change 142
    analyze data 144
    collect data 144
    evaluate effectiveness 145
    implement change 144
    objectives 142
    plan the change strategy 144
    stages 142
        moving 142
        refreezing 143
        unfreezing 142
Planning and organization of clinical learning experiences 169
    assignments 171
    criteria used in selecting clinical area for student experience 169
    general plan for learning-based 169
    general principles in selecting learning experiences 169
    orientation of students to clinical area 171
    planning activities 170
    planning students experiences in cooperation with the head nurse and team leaders 170
Planning learning experiences 151
Planning process 55
    activities of planning 56
        elements in planning 58
        strategic planning 56
        tactical planning 56
    objectives 55
    purpose of planning 56
Power 5
    types 5
        coercive power 6
        expert power 6
        legitimate power 6
        referent power 6
        reward power 6
Professional health service departments 78
    accident and emergency department 80
        operating theater 80
    medical department 78
    nursing department 78
    outpatient department 80
    paramedical departments 78
        dietary department 79

laboratory 78
pharmacy department 79
physical medicine and rehabilitation department 79
radiology department 79

Q

Qualities of a leader 34
  credibility and forward thinking 34
    advocacy 36
    professionalism 36
  interpersonal relationships 34
  managerial abilities 34
  temperament 34
Qualities of a measuring instruments 178
  content validity 178
  equilibrium 179
  equity 179
  objectivity 179
  practicability 179
  predictive validity 179
  reliability 179
  specificity 179
  validity 178
Quality assurance 125
  approaches to quality assurance 126
    outcome element 125
    process element 126
    structural element 126
  steps 126
    assign responsibility 127
    data collection 127
    delineate scope of care 127
    determining criteria 127
    evaluating performance 128
    identify important aspects of care 127
    monitoring and feedback 129
    problem identification 128
    problem solution 128
    setting standards 126
Quality assurance (QA) 124
Quality assurance methods 129
  nursing audit 129
  patient care profiles analysis 129
  patient satisfaction 129
  peer review 129
  quality circles 129

R

Records 133
  kinds 133
  purposes 133

Reports 137
  kinds 137
    accuracy 139
    confidentiality 139
    oral 137
    permanence 139
    written 138
  purposes 137
Responsibility for conducting staff development programs 123
Role of assessment in the educational process 182
Role of nurse manager 89
  levels of management 90
    first level management 90
    middle level management 90
    upper/top level management 90
  objectives 89
  roles and responsibilities 89
Role of the nurse manager in staff development 123

S

Scheduling/duty roster 102
  guide to compiling duty roster 104
    part A 104
    part B 105
  objectives 102
  principles in planning the duty roster 102
    continuity 103
    cost effectiveness 103
    coverage 103
    flexibility 103
    stability 103
  purposes of scheduling 102
  scheduling policies 103
  steps in planning duty roster 103
Staff development 118
  objectives 118
  types 118
    induction training 119
    in-service education 119
    orientation 119
Staff development model 119
  orientation program 120
    advantages 120
    objective 120
  programs for staff development 120
  skill training program 121
    key behaviors 121
    objectives 121
Staff motivation 113
  job dissatisfaction 114
  motivation theories 114
  need for motivation 113
  objectives 113

Staffing 98
    factors which affect staffing 98
        client factors 99
        personnel factors 99
        philiosophy and objectives 98
        work environment factors 99
    objectives 98
    patient care needs 99
        calculation of the required number of staffing 100
        direct patient care 100
        indirect care 100
        time standard 100
    staffing process 99
Steps in management process 7
    objectives 7
Strategic planning 57
Strategies/methods of clinical teaching 173
    counseling 177
    demonstration 173
    evaluation 177
    nurse rounds and clinical rounds 173
    orientation 173
    pre-and postconferences 173
        objectives 174
    ward staff meetings 175
    ward teaching/case study presentation 174
Symptoms of motivated nurses 116
Systems analysis 67
    basic principles of system approach 68
        advantages 68
        disadvantages 68
Systems theory 65
    feedback and control 67
    objectives 65
    types of systems 65
        closed systems 65
        open systems 65

T

Taylor's monistic theory 114
Test construction 182
Test item 182
    types 183
        limited choice items 183
        open ended 183
Time management 37
    importance 37
    objectives 37
    principles 37
        daily planning and scheduling 38
        delegation 39
        evaluation 41
        goal setting 38
        personal organization and self-discipline 39
        plan strategies 39
        respecting time 41
        schedule office visits 40
        schedule paper work 41
        selection of staff 37
        setting priorities 38
        time analysis 41
        transition time 40
        use meetings effectively 41
Transformational leadership 26
Trends in nursing curriculum development 154
    classification 154
        general educational trends 155
        science and technological trends 155
        social trends 155
        trends in nursing education and nursing practice 156
        trends in the health care system 156

U

Unit plan 197